Praise for *Never Let Them See You Sweat*

"Dr. Leigh Vinocur combines her personal journey with science-backed strategies in a way that's enlightening, funny, and deeply inspiring. She offers practical tools to reduce stress, build resilience, and thrive in life, love, and career—all while reminding us to give ourselves a break when we need it. Her comprehensive guide is relatable, empowering, and truly indispensable."
— **Dr. Shikha Jain, FACP, University of Illinois, Founder and Board Member of Women in Medicine®, and CEO and Founder of Women in Medicine Summit™**

"Enlightening, funny, and deeply inspiring. Dr. Vinocur masterfully blends her personal journey with cutting-edge science, offering not just a roadmap to manage stress but a powerful guide to thrive in the face of it."
— **Bill Donovan, President of the Pritikin Longevity Center**

"Dr. Leigh Vinocur provides practical and science-backed strategies to reduce stress, build resilience, achieve great things—and know when to give yourself a break! Her comprehensive guide covers so many aspects of life, love, and career that every reader will find it highly relatable and ultimately indispensable."
— **Melanie Notkin, Founder of Savvy Auntie, and Author of *OTHER-HOOD: Modern Women Finding a New Kind of Happiness***

"Dr. Leigh Vinocur's book challenges conventional wisdom about stress. While rooted in robust scientific research, her funny and personal anecdotes, wry humor, and compassionate insights make the book both informative and enjoyable. Through her personal stories, she provides practical techniques to readers with tools to reinterpret their stress response. It is a compelling and highly recommended read for anyone looking to better manage stress in their lives and enhance their overall quality of life."
— **Dr. Steven Sobelman-Author, Licensed Psychologist and Emeritus Psychology Professor, Loyola University of Maryland**

"Dr. Leigh's delivers a fun, yet highly researched and informative, book about stress and how to alleviate it—even harness it. Her sometimes humorous climb up the medical and media ladder shows her own ability to *Never Let Them See You Sweat*. You'll love the chapter about "Vanity's Little Secret!" I recommend this book for anyone, particularly women, who aspire to go beyond their stress while pursuing their best selves."

— Dr. Mike Dow, Best-Selling Author of *The Brain Fog Fix*

"Dr. Leigh's sense of humor shines through as she reveals some of the most stressful stages in her life. Then she provides an array of techniques, which are backed by science, to relieve stress. I love her "best investment of her life," a bathtub where she literally soaks the stress away.

— Dr. Skyler Hamilton, Author of *Empower Your Child to Heal*

"In this engaging and useful book, Dr. Leigh Vinocur takes on the dual role of trusted physician and candid friend, looking us in the eye and telling us when we're overreacting and what to do when stress has already gotten the best of us (which is way too often). Drawing on scientific research, she delivers actionable advice paired with easy-to-implement tips and concise takeaways at the end of each chapter. This breezy yet meaty book is especially empowering for women. She highlights the vital roles of self-confidence and self-advocacy, weaving in her own laugh-out-loud moments and heartfelt stories to remind us that we're all in this together."

— Kim Rittenberg, Former Media Executive turned Award-Winning Founder of Henry Street Media

Never Let Them
See You Sweat

Never Let Them See You Sweat

How Science Can Help Us Harness Stress for Success

By Leigh Vinocur, MD, MS

HAMILTON BOOKS

HAMILTON BOOKS
Bloomsbury Publishing Inc, 1385 Broadway, New York, NY 10018, USA
Bloomsbury Publishing Plc, 50 Bedford Square, London, WC1B 3DP, UK
Bloomsbury Publishing Ireland, 29 Earlsfort Terrace, Dublin 2, D02 AY28, Ireland

BLOOMSBURY, HAMILTON BOOKS and the Diana logo are trademarks of
Bloomsbury Publishing Plc

First published in the United States of America 2025

Library of Congress Cataloging-in-Publication Data Available

Library of Congress Control Number: 2025938137

ISBN: 978-0-7618-7436-2 (pbk : alk. paper)
ISBN: 978-0-76187-437-9 (ebook)

Typeset by Deanta Global Publishing Services, Chennai, India

For product safety related questions contact productsafety@bloomsbury.com.

To find out more about our authors and books visit www.bloomsbury.com and sign up
for our newsletters.

Dedication

I dedicate this book to my mother, Lynn. She was my best friend, my cheerleader, my confidante, and my "enabler" in the best of ways. Her unconditional, unwavering love and support has enabled me to do all the things I ever dreamed of doing. This has propelled me throughout my life to unabashedly try and believe that I could do anything I put my mind to!

And I am also dedicating this book to all the unbelievable women I have had the good fortune to meet and befriend throughout all the different phases of my life. To my childhood friends: bestie Denise; Susan and Mary Kate; my college friend, Gail; my medical school friends, Suzy and Amy; and my adult friends, Flo, Nancy, Elaine, Lorraine, Risa and Lisa. You all show me not only how important female friendships are, but you also inspire me every day.

*Thank you all for just being who you are, and
I hope this book will inspire others.*

Contents

Preface

I wrote this book for you. So often women come up to me and ask me how I do it all. They think I have it all together because I've had a successful 30-plus year career in medicine, even a pioneer in some cases; I was the first female resident doctor in a urology residency program—and do I have stories from then! I've been a medical educator on and off the screen, chief medical officer and medical director in the nutraceutical and biotech industry, a cannabis medical consultant, emergency physician, and clinical trial director among other professional positions; I've published studies, lay articles, contributed to numerous national media outlets; I've served as spokesperson for the American College of Emergency Physicians; and I have appeared regularly as a television medical analyst on *NewsNation*, HLN, *The Dr. Oz Show*, *The Today Show*, Fox News, CNN, and others.

While women think I never have doubts about myself, just like anyone else, I have my own fair share of meltdowns, freak-outs, trials, tribulations, and stressors that have caused occasional anxiety. Growing up as a perfectionist I developed an affinity for stress I would overcompensate for—or brace for with superstitious routines. Throughout motherhood, medical school, and subsequent career reinventions, I've found that stress can motivate, or it can demoralize.

As a doctor, I was trained not to show stress, so I've had to roll with the punches many times and find time to relieve stress in my own ways. There's no doubt in my mind that every stage in life has unique stressors, and each one has its own challenges—some more difficult than others—and some might even call for professional help.

But I want to let you know that doubts, stresses, and imposter syndrome— which I've experienced even while writing this book—do not have to define us or hold us back! Throughout my life I have met so many wonderful women who sell themselves short, starting with my beloved mother. She was one of the smartest women I ever knew. During her school days in the 1940s, she would skip class to read books in her grandmother's attic. Neighbors would call her grandmother and say they'd seen her walking across the street with her head in a book again. She was also the kid reading another book inside her schoolbook during class. Her teachers, and even her parents, somewhat wrote her off. After all, women back then were just expected to marry a doctor, not become one. That is why everyone was so surprised when she scored the highest score in her high school on the standardized tests and college entrance exams. She really could have done anything she wanted with her life. But after two years of college, she met my dad, an older doctor, and her parents pushed her to marry. She quickly had me at 19 years old! After that she chose to push me and my brother to be all we could.

I will mention her often in this book because she was my number-one stress reliever and confidence booster; her support allowed me to try new things and not fear failure as much. My hope is to use this book to do the same for you.

Dr. Leigh

Acknowledgements

I would like to thank and acknowledge David Jahr, whose help, guidance and organization with this book has been invaluable! And to Popi Edi, who was devoted to my mom and always there for her, even to the very end. I must also thank TonyD, the love of my life, whose love and support keep me going in every new adventure we take on. And to my son Max who has been an inspiration to me since he was a toddler, his wit, his brains and his love keep me going even when I thought I couldn't… I love you to infinity and beyond!

Introduction

After watching my second husband drive off with all his belongings, I slumped down in a corner of our walk-in closet. The stress and anxiety from our failed marriage combined with the realization that he was actually gone gave me plenty of reason to start a pity party. After all, this was my second failed marriage, and perhaps I had a teensy share of the blame for its demise. I sat there feeling sorry for myself as I watched him from the window drive down our long private drive. Then out of the corner of my eye, I noticed a lone hanger, still swinging on his side of the empty closet.

Suddenly, I realized there might be a bright side. I got up and rushed down the stairs, opened the spare closet, and gathered up all my winter clothes. Finally, I had enough room in my bedroom closet for *both* seasons of clothing. I may have been losing a husband, but I was gaining a closet! This was a of a bit tongue-in-cheek revelation but finding the humor in most situations has always saved me. And I did often tell myself that in bleak situations, it is all in how you look things.

That's how I embarked on my next adventure in life—life as a single mom. While I don't mean to make light of divorce, it doesn't do any good to dwell on it either. This approach also helped me address the stress and anxiety in new ways. I believed the faster I could move forward into the next phase of life, the sooner I could relieve my stress about it all. And my ex and I remain on friendly terms for our son.

As an emergency physician and television medical analyst, I've become an expert in harnessing stress and anxiety. These professions rank right up there as the most stressful, so I've learned a thing or two about hiding, relieving, and harnessing stress. Broadcast journalism and emergency medicine are actually very similar in that you must be ready for anything at a moment's notice. Whether a life-threatening emergency is coming into the ER or you receive a call from a station looking for a medical expert to speak on break-ing news with medical implications, you never want them to see you sweat!

While deep down I am an optimist, I tend to wear a pessimist's cloak. I think and expect the worst in any given situation, which has served me well as an emergency physician—making sure I rule out your worst, potentially life-threatening, diagnosis first. But somehow, even when things seem their darkest, I ultimately believe that it will all work out for the best.

Much of my optimism comes from my mom—she was a real Pollyanna—but also from my spirituality, also instilled in me by my mom. She could always find the good in a situation I was worried about and then unburden me of my stress and anxiety by telling me how it would all work out in the end. Now as a mom myself, living without her, I see how in unburdening me, she probably burdened herself with my worries. I was always anxious and wondering if I would be able to continue without her support—she was such a wonderful mother, mentor, and role model—but I see now that she prepared me to live and eventually thrive without her.

My emergency medical training has also taught me to triage my stresses. Emergency physicians are taught to triage patients; in fact, that is how emer-gency departments function. They do not work on a first-come, first-serve basis. Thankfully, you don't have to take a number with a heart attack and get behind the guy with the paper cut! Triage comes from the French derivation, "to sort." Patients are categorized to determine who has a life- or limb-threat-ening injury or illness and then seen according to the severity of their issue.

Nowhere is triage more important than in responding to a mass casualty event, which we are unfortunately now seeing all too often with escalating gun violence in the US. And this is how, out of necessity, I learned to triage my stresses for survival and success. In a mass causality situation,[1] doctors and emergency medical services must make quick decisions about who to help first. They assess who has the least severe injuries, those who will sur-vive no matter what, then determine who has the most severe injuries, the patients who will die no matter what is done. It is the patients in the middle that will survive with interventions.

In my life, I try to let go of the stresses or worries that will not change no matter what I do. For example, at one point when my mother was dying and I was caring for her, I had to come to the realization that we could not change her outcome. I had to let go of the fear of losing her so that I could spend the quality time with her in whatever time she had left.

I also let go of the minor worries and annoyances that won't hurt or affect me in the long term—things like annoying people who cut in front of you in bumper-to-bumper traffic. I recognize that it's the worries and stress in the middle that I have some control over; so those are the stresses that I focus on.

Even without the emergency-physician training for mass casualties, my mom had this approach down pat. When I would confide in her about my stress or worries, she would say, "Really Leigh, is that worth having a heart attack or getting cancer over? Let it go, baby."

Ironically, I am writing this book at one of the most stressful times in my life, second only to caring for my dying mother. Right now, I fully understand the term *sandwich generation*. Although I don't have young kids at home, for the past two years I acted as the primary caregiver for a 98-year-old friend with dementia and blindness (who just passed away). I was also caring for my dad, who had been living with me for over a year while he got multiple reconstructive surgeries. My son also still calls on me daily (as I did with my mom) for support through his PhD program. Of course, like all moms, I don't know anything and am not qualified to give advice, so I need to just listen. I find that daughters are much different than sons in that respect. We also just lost my stepdaughter suddenly at 41 years old, despite her cancer treatments going well.

That brings me to the reason I am writing this book now. The pandemic years, with the divisive politics and rancor that ensued, and that still exist today even more than ever, tested everyone—and not all of us have fully rebounded. The constant stress, grief, and loss has been felt by all of us and has caused record numbers of people feeling burned out with stress and/or mental health issues. Life continues to pile more on every day, in that I know I am not alone.

In my specialty of emergency medicine, we see severe burnout. I still see so many colleagues bewildered from the frontline fight with COVID-19. In an article I wrote for *MedPageToday*[2] I described the unprecedented stress and burnout my fellow emergency medicine colleagues faced during the pandemic, which still lingers today with our overcrowded, overtaxed emergency rooms around the country.

And it isn't just physicians; one study suggested the mental health of the average middle-aged American has recently seen the worst decline in decades.[3] Mental health needs to be a priority for everyone. But stress is not *all* bad. Stress is an evolutionary biological response designed to support and protect us. It is part of our survival instinct. Think of the Stone Age; we needed to develop a keen mechanism to survive life-or-death situations while hunting or being hunted. It is our fight-or-flight response. During prehistoric time, this was particularly helpful when running from a saber-tooth tiger. But that life-or-death response is not needed as often when you're an accountant sitting in an office.

Small amounts of intermittent stress get you going and keep you in tip-top shape to act when needed. Think of the athlete standing in the racing blocks before the gun goes off; they need these short bursts of adrenaline from stress to function in top form. However, chronic high levels of stress that serve no purpose take their toll and wear down our bodies physically and emotionally.

Unfortunately, stress is unavoidable. There's no such thing as living stress-free. Our mind and body are designed to recognize stress and react to it, while maintaining our homeostasis. Our immune system is a great example; it has an adaptive ability to recognize threats like oxidative stress, bacteria, and viruses, and learn how to mount an offensive to fight these off the next time they encounter them. Stress is 100 percent natural, even good for you sometimes.

That means we don't always have to turn to medications to "manage" stress. I believe we must learn to face our fears, become resilient, cope with what's freaking us out, and become better people from it. We can harness stress for the greater good of ourselves and futures. This is why I'm writing this book. I've had a career with personal highs and lows that made me cry and cringe and brought me to tears with laughter. I hope you find my story relatable and my evidence-based suggestions to be a relief, because it is possible to harness stress for success and to produce a positive outcome.

In these pages, I am going to open up about various moments in my life where I had to stare down stress. I've been beside myself and tried many ways to calm down. Throughout my lifetime, I have learned the dos and don'ts for handling stress and anxiety, which I'll share in here and hopefully give you a giggle. Laughter is, after all, the best medicine to relieve stress, and that's no joke. One researcher found that laughter can mitigate the effects of stress by decreasing stress-making hormones. Laughter can decrease serum levels of stress hormones such as cortisol and adrenaline, indicating a reversal of the stress response.[4]

I'll also discuss what actually happens to the brain and body when stress and anxiety occur—what makes them crippling as panic sets in. I'll suggest cathartic ways to reduce stress that may save you from sitting in a therapist's chair, not that there's anything wrong with that. There are times when it's absolutely necessary to get professional help to unravel your fears, hurts, and resentments that boil over into anxiety and depression. I'll discuss research about different medical treatments that show promise.

But sometimes the best thing for me to do is bake and decorate a cake. There's something therapeutic about the process that takes my mind off the cares of the world by focusing on transforming simple ingredients into a delicious, and dare I say, beautiful work of art. Science is behind me on this too. One study found that people doing culinary activities not only obtain pure happiness and relaxation but can draw wider inferences about their life by realizing their own potential. That is probably why baking took off during the psychologically challenging COVID-19 lockdown days.[5]

Maybe psychiatrists should prescribe a new recipe instead of anti-anxiety medication! That's just one example of how I've learned to harness stress to create something amazing, but there's much more to uncover in this book. By learning how to harness your stress, you can turn it into success. You can turn it into resilience. You can reduce it, steward it, and achieve something great. So, keep turning the pages. I hope to crack you up and energize you to mobilize your stress instead of letting it knock you down. I hope to empower you the way my mother did for me, to let you know that you are capable of handling anything; together we can harness our stress for success!

Part I

SPEAKING FROM EXPERIENCE

Chapter 1

The Physiology of Stress

Race day arrived. As schools of runners, jumpers, throwers, and pole vault-ers competed under the sun at my high school track and field meet, anxiety started running through my veins. The 100-meter dash was coming up, and I was one of the racers. Even though I was somewhat fast, I had one of the most common knee problems seen in adolescent girls, subluxing patellas, due to years of playing sports while growing up. My kneecaps were unstable and would move laterally out of joint in certain positions and with certain activities.[1]

While stretching and warming up for the race, my nerves got me thinking of a way to fix my knee in place. Instead of asking my coach for help, I took matters into my own hands and struggled to pull a tight ankle brace over my knee for stability. My crazy thinking was that I could push hard while sprint-ing and not worry about my kneecaps tracking out of the joint.

"On your mark. Get set. *Bang!*" The gun went off.

I started running, if you could call it that. I was the opposite of a graceful sprinter. Every time I tried to bend my knee, the too-tight brace snapped my leg straight again, essentially making me limp and hobble throughout the running stride, like a lame horse that needed to be put down (not that I would ever condone that). I could see the look on my coach's face: a mix of wonder-ment and disbelief at what the heck was going on with me. And of course, no surprise, I came in last place. The moral of this story, besides not wearing an ankle brace on your knee (unless your thighs are really skinny), is that some-times we overcompensate for stress and make matters worse.

Before we talk about relieving stress and anxiety, it's important to under-stand why we experience it in the first place. Because stress does serve a physiologic purpose. Stress is a survival instinct, and as we will see, it can be harnessed. It keeps us alert and aware of danger, focused on a task, and even

3

motivated. So, it's important to know that stress is not a character flaw or personal weakness. It's natural and 100 percent normal and an evolutionary response we developed to keep us safe.

Our brain and nervous system instruct our body to produce hormones that help us cope when acute stress arrives. The adrenal glands release hormones, including adrenaline, noradrenaline, and cortisol; this is often referred to as the fight-or-flight response, which is more accurately described as the fight-or-flight-or-freeze response.

Stress is a biological chain reaction meant to support and protect us. During prehistoric times, this fight-or-flight response was the evolutionary adaptation we developed to help us survive life-or-death situations while hunting and gathering. When facing a life-threatening situation, our body activates the autonomic nervous system (ANS) with this response so we can either fight like a badger or run like a deer. However, the stress response can stop us in our tracks or make us faint, which may seem counterintuitive, but some evolutionary biologists theorize that, in animals, freezing may offer more time to assess the situation for eventual escape.[2]

Nevertheless, our ANS controls involuntary activities as well as our internal organs. The ANS is comprised of the parasympathetic nervous system, which controls body functions at rest, like digestion, and the sympathetic nervous system, which prepares the body for the fight-or-flight response.[3]

Luckily today, most humans rarely need to flee from predators, yet life is full of stressors, and even during happy occasions we can feel tension building up. Our stressors come in the form of social, financial, and emotional varieties. In fact, stress and anxiety are among the most searched-for topics regarding mental health. Events over recent years, especially the COVID-19 pandemic and the ongoing political climate, has highlighted this even more. Americans are feeling added pressures from these difficult and uncertain times. Even before the pandemic a global Gallup Poll found that Americans are among the most stressed-out and unhappy people in the world.[4]

But our protective stress response is supposed to be self-limited and temporary. After the cause of stress is over, the body can rebalance so that we can feel calm again. Let's take a closer look at what is happening in our bodies.

OUR PHYSIOLOGICAL RESPONSE

What happens in our brains and bodies when we experience a stressful event? It begins in an area in the brain called the amygdala, where our emotions and responses to threatening stimuli are regulated and processed; the amygdala works to help us detect real threats and activate the appropriate fearful responses to dangers.[5] It then sends signals to the hypothalamus to stimulate the ANS—specifically the sympathetic nervous system—causing your adrenal glands to release adrenaline and cortisol. These hormones in turn prepare the body for its fight-or-flight response with the following physiologic changes:

- Breathing speeds up and small airways dilate to get more oxygen into our system.
- The heart starts beating faster to pump blood and oxygen to our muscles in preparation for fight-or-flight.
- Senses are heightened, hearing sharpens—the way animals' ears perk up when they sense danger—and our pupils dilate, letting more light in and increasing our peripheral vision to look for escape routes if fleeing.
- Blood gets diverted from internal organs, like our digestive system, and sent to our muscles in preparation to run or fight.
- This response can even dampen pain perception in anticipation for our need to fight.

But this response is only meant to last 30 minutes or so, while the imminent threat is still present.[6]

Chronic stress causes these hormones to remain active and circulating for sustained periods of time; the effects on the brain and body can lead to several physical, psychological, cognitive, and behavioral problems. Therefore, we need to learn to manage our stress to avoid detrimental effects to our health and well-being—because over time, it will take a toll on our physical and mental health.[7]

Studies have found that people under stress who harbor anger, resentment, and negative emotions are three times more likely to develop premature heart disease and have a five-times greater chance of having a heart attack.[8] Research also suggests that chronic stress can affect our immune system, whether it is susceptibility to developing infections, autoimmune diseases, or even an increased cancer risk.[9]

This immune dysfunction can also lead to chronic inflammation, believed to cause dysfunction and injury to the lining of our blood vessels, with plaque buildup triggering clots. Constriction of these blood vessels can also increase risk for heart attack or stroke.[10] Chronic inflammation is also associated with a whole host of other diseases such as cancer, diabetes mellitus, chronic kidney disease, and autoimmune and neurodegenerative disorders.

Over time, chronic stress from the competing demands of our work, finances, and home life can not only contribute to heart disease and high blood pressure, but neuroscientists have also found that the brain structure is altered by chronic exposure to cortisol. That is why stress is a major contributing factor to anxiety, depression, and even addiction.

And the mind-body connection is real. People dealing with chronic stress often see it manifest in a variety of physical signs and symptoms. These include headache, heart palpitations, high blood pressure, shortness of breath, muscle and back aches, clenched jaw with teeth grinding, indigestion, abdominal pain and bloating, constipation, diarrhea, fatigue, insomnia, weight gain or loss, skin problems, problems with concentrating and memory, as well as loss of libido, just to name a few.

PHYSICIANS ARE AT A GREATER RISK

The pandemic magnified the constant stress that my emergency physician colleagues and I have dealt with for years. Not only has this led to burnout but clinicians are also leaving medicine in droves. Physicians also have one of the highest rates of suicide of any profession. Male doctors die by suicide at a rate that is 40 percent higher than the general population. Female doctors die by suicide at a rate 130 percent higher than the general population.[11]

Emergency docs are faced with life-or-death decisions daily and expected to perform perfectly. It's important that we remain calm and be strong and decisive when caring for our patients. The irony is that doctors also believe they cannot, and must not, reveal having any stress, or their own reputation and career will be at stake.

In medical school, we were encouraged, and even trained, to "never let them see you sweat" and to be ready for anything. We put patient concerns ahead of ourselves, often to our own detriment. We are faulted for showing vulnerability and therefore do not ask for help.

As doctors, we faced stress, and grief, at work and especially early during the pandemic. We tried to remain isolated from our homes and our support systems to protect family members; this only added to the anxiety and depression. As emergency physicians, we try to compartmentalize all the suffering we see, but we are human, and it affects us all.

Emergency medicine is particularly stressful and known for high burnout rates. As emergency physicians we feel the need to be superhuman while on shift, but many colleagues have admitted to me that the hardest part of the day is when they finish their shifts and they are alone, processing the day's pressure, stress, and grief. The toll our days take on us may not manifest until later down the road. For some, it can be too much to bear.

Emergency physicians were mourning the loss of one of our best and brightest, Lorna Breen, MD, who left us by suicide in April 2020. I fear there will be many more tragedies, unless we break the stigma of mental illness and end the idea that for a physician, seeking treatment is taboo. Physicians in all specialties are reluctant to reach out for mental health help, even in the best of times. Many of us fear that seeking treatment could jeopardize our career. Questions from some hospital credentialing and medical licensing boards can be worded with sweeping statements that imply receiving treatment for a mental health condition would be an impairment that affects our capacity to practice. This approach may go beyond the intent of the Americans with Disabilities Act, and it is understandable that physicians are reluctant to answer the types of loaded questions on applications.

Physicians, just like everyone else, face normal pressures such as a difficult divorce, family issues with children acting out, and the death of a loved one, any of which could reasonably require a little help in the form of counseling or medication. It is unreasonable to expect a physician to absorb and handle these issues themselves while others can seek counseling or care. And it's even worse that we would feel forced to ignore or downplay these stressors.

It is tragically ironic that we act as vocal advocates for the mental health needs of our patients while we forgo treatment ourselves and hide our own human frailty. The status quo must change.

The American College of Emergency Physicians and many other medical associations are fighting to protect the health professionals responsible for millions of lives. My fellow physicians should be able to seek appropriate mental healthcare without fear of reprisal. Credentialing authorities should encourage physicians to prioritize their mental health. Doctors are human too. We should be able to get the same mental healthcare as anyone else, without feeling like we are risking our jobs.

Thankfully, the American College of Emergency Physicians and the Dr. Lorna Breen Foundation worked with Congress to enact the Dr. Lorna Breen Health Care Provider Protection Act (HR 1667), which was passed in the House and Senate unanimously (a miracle in itself). It's aimed at helping to "improve mental and behavioral health among health care providers"[12] and to reduce and prevent suicide, burnout, and mental and behavioral health conditions among health care professionals."[13]

While I'm going to outline the many ways that I have found to relieve and even harness stress, there are times when the chemical imbalances in our brain and body require professional attention or pharmaceutical intervention. And there is absolutely nothing wrong with this. The worst thing you can do is ignore the problem.

ENDOCANNABI—WHAT?

Here's another physiological system that many people, and even most physicians, are not that aware of despite the critical role it plays in maintaining homeostasis in our body. It's called our endocannabinoid system (ECS).

In 2008, I was on faculty at the University of Maryland School of Medicine, and I was talking to a colleague and researcher about his work studying endocannabinoid levels in stressed rats.

"What word did you use? Endo-what?" I asked. "Do you mean we have internal cannabinoids like enkephalins and endorphins that are analogous to our internal opioids?" I was stunned that I had been practicing medicine for over 15 years at that point and I had never heard of the ECS.

This system is made up of our own internal cannabinoid compounds and their receptors. I was just blown away by its apparent role in our health! The more I learned, the more intrigued I was about this topic, and what we do, and don't know about how it works. I started reading everything I could find on the subject. The basic science research was fascinating. I had no idea how integral it was to our *homeostasis*, a term that means maintaining a stable functioning and equilibrium of our biologic system.

The ECS is an internal neuro-modulating system ingrained in our evolutionary development; most vertebrate animals (animals with backbones) but even down to the invertebrate sea squirts and hydras, have parts of this essential system that's critical for survival, allowing them to adapt to their environment.[14]

Our ECS receptors, called cannabinoid receptor 1 and 2 (CB1 and CB2),[15] were first discovered in 1988. Then the first endocannabinoid (eCB), which fit into those receptors, was isolated and discovered in 1992 by Dr. Raphael Mechoulem.[16] He was the first person to identify the intoxicating compound tetrahydrocannabinol (THC) in cannabis back in 1964.[17] This biological regulatory system modulates our nervous, endocrine, and immune systems to help maintain the function, health, and stability of these systems.

When Dr. Mechoulem discovered the first internal cannabinoid compound, called N-arachidonoylethanolamine, he later dubbed it *Anandamide* because the root word *ananda* is the Sanskrit word for bliss. It is our bliss molecule. Then in 1995, scientists discovered the second main endocannabinoid molecule, 2-Arachidonoylglycerol, called 2AG for short. These are the two main internal cannabinoid compounds our body synthesizes on demand during stressful times. However, we have now discovered many more endocannabinoids that our body synthesizes as well.

The ECS affects virtually every function and physiological system in our body. Its broad role regulates homeostasis with every stimulus we get, both internally and externally. In our central nervous system (CNS), which is comprised of our brain and spinal cord, it regulates our brain cognition, motor control, emotional responses, and motivated behaviors. It also has a role in our body affecting our immune system, our peripheral and autonomic nervous system, as well as the gastrointestinal nervous system.

Virtually every physiologic function in our bodies has been linked to our ECS, which helps us maintain and stabilize our health and address dysfunction during stress. In the CNS, the ECS affects behaviors such as cognition, eating, sleeping, memory, and pain relief. The endocannabinoids (eCB) are synthesized on demand as needed to modulate our nervous system at times of stress, at the nerve junctions, called synapses, all throughout our body.

Our eCBs are widespread, ubiquitous, and versatile signaling molecules that interact not only with our cannabinoid receptors, CB1 and CB2, but they also modulate many other neurotransmitters within our nervous system. For example, they affect our levels of serotonin, the neurotransmitter related to anxiety, happiness, and mood, which is also the target for anti-anxiety and anti-depression medications called selective serotonin reuptake inhibitors (SSRI). They affect dopamine, one of the "feel good" neurotransmitters in the reward center of our brain, which affects mood as well as movement, memory, and focus. They also modulate norepinephrine, the neurotransmitter involved in the alertness and arousal in our fight-or-flight response, but also affect mood and ability to concentrate and has been the target of another category of antidepressants know as serotonin-norepinephrine reuptake inhibitors (SNRI).

The famous endocannabinoid researcher Dr. Vincenzo Di Marzo stated, "The endocannabinoid system is essential to life, and it relates messages that affect how we relax, eat, sleep, forget and protect."[18]

The ECS is so essential to our normal functioning that another famous cannabis researcher, Dr. Ethan Russo, describes in several published papers the concept of clinical endocannabinoid deficiency (CECD); he asserts that difficult treatment-resistant conditions such as fibromyalgia, irritable bowel syndrome, and even migraines, might be due to a dysfunction or deficiency of our endocannabinoids.[19, 20] Recent studies in children with autism spectrum disorder found lower levels of endocannabinoids.[21] In fact, another study actually correlated how severe these children were on the spectrum by just looking at their anandamide levels.[22]

Conditions like epilepsy have also been found to be associated with endocannabinoid dysfunction; a study showed reduced levels of anandamide in the brains of people who were newly diagnosed with untreated seizure disorder.[23]

We need our endocannabinoid system to calm and dampen the over-excitatory signaling and activity in our nervous system, caused by many different stressors, including anxiety—and that is how it plays a role in our mental health. The bottom line is the healthier our ECS, the better able we should be to handle stresses.

We are only beginning to learn about the intersection of health and disease and how our endocannabinoid system relates to that, as well as how external phytocannabinoids (*phyto*, meaning plant) found in the cannabis plant, among others, may be used to treat disease that might be the result of an endocannabinoid system dysfunction. This is why, perhaps, many of these difficult-to-treat medical conditions such as autism and drug-resistant seizure disorders do often respond to cannabis as a medical therapy. But that is a vast topic for my next book!

It was learning and reading about this fascinating, relatively new, field in medical science, years ago, that pushed me toward another career challenge and journey. I decided to get one of the country's first master's degrees from the University of Maryland School of Pharmacy in medical cannabis science and therapeutics. And later in the book, we will look at the scientific research that explores the use of cannabis and the phytocannabinoids in the treatment of anxiety and depression.

For now, the primary message of this chapter is to allow yourself to feel stress. It's a normal biological response designed to protect us. Since we rarely have a need to run for our lives, we need to understand how to address the psychology of stress and anxiety. In future chapters, I'll give you ways to reduce and refocus stress and anxiety. Next, however, let's take a brief look at the psychology of stress to fully appreciate where it's coming from.

Key Takeaways

- Short-term stress is a normal, protective physiological response to external dangers.
- Chronic stress is the problem that contributes to physical and mental health illnesses.
- We have an internal stress-modulating system called the endocannabinoid system; however, its dysfunction can lead to medical problems that are hard to treat with conventional medications.

Chapter 2

The Psychology of Stress

After an episode of freezing rain, typical of winter in Maryland since it typically does not get quite cold enough to just snow, I walked down our long driveway hill, dragging the trash behind me with my beloved dog in tow on her leash. As I looked for areas of asphalt that appeared to be free of ice, I mistook a sheet of black ice for a clear spot, and *whoosh*, my right foot slipped, sending both legs up into the sky.

Midair, I twisted and landed on my left knee, which promptly shot my patella—kneecap—to the side (something that has caused me trouble for ages) and landed me on my ass. The trash cans toppled and emptied themselves on the driveway as I winced in pain. I had not had a subluxation (partial dislocation) of my left kneecap this bad since medical school when I had been running to a code blue in the ER and ended up slipping on the freshly mopped floor for which maintenance had yet to put up the warning signs.

Having just watched a news report about a remarkable German shepherd that ran across state lines to get help for its unconscious owner in a car crash, I yelled, "Nellie! Go home and get help." But she didn't move, just stared at me with a look that seemed to say, "So, are we going on the walk or not?" So much for her Lassie moment! Fortunately, my son heard me and came out to help me to my feet and complete the disastrous chore.

I decided to see my orthopedic surgeon, which I usually don't do for this type of injury because my knee often heals on its own with rest. But I wanted to ask about a steroid shot so I could continue my obsessive Peloton racing with other old-fart-60-year-olds looking for glory on the leaderboard and to maintain my weight. He greeted me with, "What's up? You never come in, even when I tell you check back," to which I responded he should be happy to see me, as my bad knees are like an annuity for him; they just keep giving and giving. Despite my begging to get back in the game on my bike, he told me the pain was there for a reason, and he didn't want me back on the bike for a couple of weeks.

Deflated on my way out, mad that I could not continue working out, I started feeling sorry for myself. I was lamenting about my probable weight gain over the next few weeks as well as stressing about how my mental health might suffer without this outlet. Then, I saw a young woman shuffling past me with a walker. She had an above-the-knee amputation on her right leg and wore a prosthesis for a below-the-knee amputation on her left side. I immediately felt like an idiot, realizing how trivial my complaints and problems were compared to what she was enduring. I instantly started feeling grateful for what I had. I told myself, *Thank God, this is just a stupid patellar subluxation.*

It dawned on me, sometimes the best cure for stress is to put a situation into perspective. A conscious decision and effort to be both grateful and empathetic can help release that stress. You see, while stress has a biological function, too much can, obviously, be harmful. Chronic stress and anxiety can have far-reaching physical effects, even leading to increased risk of disease. A quick Google Scholar search resulted in over 3.6 million published medical studies and articles linking chronic stress to physical disease.

Aside from heart disease and stroke, chronic stress can increase the risk of diabetes, cancer, and autoimmune diseases, just to name a few.[1] It can even contribute to periodontal disease[2] or susceptibility to respiratory infections like the common cold[3] in addition to being linked to premature mortality.[4]

There is also mental health and the psychological responses that we have to stress and anxiety, such as irritability, sadness, anger, mood swings, insecurity, resentment, and only seeing the negative side of things. These emotions are often skewed by our thoughts and beliefs, and our unfounded fears.

I thought my mother was the most secure, relaxed person I had ever known. She was a master at relieving my fears and stresses my entire life. When she was a young woman, and even into early middle age, she was beautiful and sexy. My mother was an actress; her stage name was Lynn Leigh Laurence—she took on the names of my brother and me. She'd get catcalls wherever we went, and my brother and I would get special gifts and favors from shopkeepers and in restaurants when we were with her. She was an eternal optimist, and a real-life Pollyanna radiating good energy, caring, and warmth that was extremely attractive.

Her second husband was 10 years younger than she (and just 10 years older than me), but they looked the same age. My mother's youthfulness was in part due to good genes, but it was also the result of taking good care of those genes, and the body that held them. For instance, she was into fitness and exercise before it became fashionable for women to go to gyms or work up a sweat.

At some point during her later middle age, my mother became very busy with, and even distracted by, our family life. Like many women, she was a complete giver, always putting herself last. She focused all her attention on my brother and me, as well as my stepdad's career as a pro golfer. We superseded any concern she had about herself and her appearance. Unlike her younger days, as a 50-something housewife, she never took a minute for herself. Inevitable weight gain followed, and those extra pounds precipitated a loss of any remaining interest in maintaining her appearance.

My mother began to claim to be "fat and happy." Perhaps she was relieved to no longer spend so much time keeping ahead of her changing body. When she would say to me, "Leigh, I hope you feel the same someday," my first thought would be, *God, I hope that never ever happens!* I tried to reignite the interest in herself she once had, but she'd just dismiss my attempts and change the subject.

I loved my mother so much and was often sad about this. She was my best friend, and I was hers, and I knew that ignoring her health could have consequences. When she became very ill, she told her oncologist, "Who needs hospice? I have Leigh to take care of me!" That made me very proud and happy, yet sad at the same time because I had to face the realization that my mom—my best friend, mentor, and idol—was going to die. It was hard for me to imagine that she really meant it when she claimed to be "fat and happy."

Before being diagnosed with cancer, my mother lost 10 pounds without trying; significant weight loss like this is one of the cardinal signs of cancer. Even though I often kill myself trying to lose 3 to 5 pounds and get deflated when I stand on the scale only to see no change, if I ever get on the scale and see I have dropped a couple of pounds more easily than I expected, the neurotic Jewish voice in my head suddenly says, *Oh my God, I must have cancer!* But we will address that self-imposed stress later in the book.

I remember my mother looking at her reflection in the mirror, grabbing her tummy, and saying, "I wish I could get rid of this." So, she *did* care, but she didn't let her appearance, nor other people's opinions of her appearance, affect her attitude. She ended up quitting acting because she didn't need outside validation the way some actors do. She was a trailblazer on self-acceptance before *body-shaming* ever became a term!

The only problem with my mother's "fat and happy" attitude was that the fat part was attributed to her poor diet and exercise habits later in life and probably contributed to her cancer and early death. We buried my mother when she was just 67, far too young, especially for a woman who had such a zest for life, and such an indefatigable sense of humor. After chemotherapy, her weight had dropped from over 180 pounds to a mere 80, and she looked at me and said, "Honey, thank God I was fat. Otherwise I would have been dead months ago from the chemo wasting!"

Attitude is so important when it comes to mental health. We are finding out more and more about how our emotions and mental health affect our physical health. Some studies have shown that being mentally healthy can be protective in aging and lower your risk of chronic diseases.[5]

The cliché, "You're only as old as you feel," may be true. But there are caveats. My dad, who died even younger than my mom at just 57 years old, said to me after his third and final cancer diagnosis (which gives you more insight into my neurotic stress and fear of getting cancer), while he was lying in his hospital, dying, "It was such a strange feeling being betrayed by my physical body, because mentally I don't feel any differently than when I was 20 years old." However, he, too, did not make the best lifestyle choices and let stress and resentment for all kinds of issues throughout his adult life eat at him. Some studies show that those with suppressed anger and anxiety that give way to hopelessness and depression might in fact be more prone to cancer.[6] Therefore, the combination of our mental attitude and healthy lifestyles choices is critical.

Because our negative emotions negatively impact both our physical and mental health, it is important to intervene and address our feelings and stressors. Studies have shown that even in healthy individuals, negative emotions have longer lasting harmful cardiovascular effects than positive emotions.[7]

My attitude is somewhere in between my chubby, happy-hippie mother's I-don't-care-what-people-think and 'I let it all out' (and by all, I mean her tush, stomach, and boobs) attitude and my neurotic Nana's (pre-Spanx) high-rise girdle suck-it-all-in and stand-up straight strictness. I don't always agree with the warm-and-fuzzy cliché of total acceptance of yourself making you beautiful. I think it could be something of the opposite. It is not self-loathing to have a never-ending drive to stay young, fit, and looking good, because it can actually improve your health. Studies have shown that looking older than your age is in fact a risk factor for poorer health.[8] We will discuss this further in Chapter 5.

As I said in the introduction, when faced with stress, we can triage. We can identify which stressors we can actually change—these are the ones to work on. I've learned that there must be some acceptance of the reality of my situation. For instance, no matter how hard I exercise and diet, my legs will never be as long as a super model's. And relinquishing myself from that, I admit, is somewhat comforting. You grow into acceptance as you age, but then again, it could just be the sheer exhaustion from crying and cursing in the dressing room mirror while trying on bathing suits that do not fit!

But seriously, we women must learn how to cut ourselves some slack. We need to stop the search to attain *the* perfect body and just focus on what we feel should be *our* perfect bodies—and let the stress of trying to look like a celebrity subside. By slowly identifying the parts of your body that you not only accept but actually like about yourself, you make yourself feel desirable. When you feel desirable, your confidence goes up and your stress goes down.

Psychologists use many different tools to measure stress; one is called the Perceived Stress Scale (PSS)[9]—one of the most widely used to measure the nonspecific perception of stress to a particular situation or time in someone's life. The 10-question survey with individual scores ranging from 0 to 40 (0 to 13 being low stress, 14 to 26 moderate, and 27 to 40 high perceived stress). It is not an absolute, but a measure of your perception of your situation. Often those perceptions begin with your thoughts, fears, and worries, despite whether others may see them as unfounded. All that really matters is that it is your perception and how you see them.

Stress can be a reaction to a fear or emotion, which begins with a thought. Therefore, it's important to identify and validate these thoughts and feelings. Later in the book, we will discuss when uncontrollable intrusive thoughts may require medical intervention, but most of us can make use of coping skills to help us harness, or even eliminate, some of the thoughts contributing to our stress levels. Sometimes it can be as simple as laughter and not taking yourself too seriously—seeing the comedy in our own reactions and situations. The beloved late comedian actor, Betty White once said, "If you take yourself lightly and don't take yourself too seriously, pretty soon you can find humor in our everyday lives. And sometimes, it can be a lifesaver." She was absolutely right!

While I was nervous about preparing for the 100-meter dash I mentioned in chapter 1, I can look back and see that I was afraid I would let the team down with my unpredictable knees. This pushed me to do something without thinking rationally. I ended up embarrassing myself, and I felt like I let the team down anyway. What could I have done differently that race day? Any number of things would have been better than putting an ankle brace on my knee. Instead, the results were hilarious, especially if you saw me run that day like a wounded gelding. But allowing everyone a good laugh at my expense helped me to diffuse the stress and anger I was feeling at myself that day. There's a little psychology behind the physiology of stress. I believe we can learn to turn stress on and off, and even learn how to benefit from it, but we must learn to identify when it all becomes too much to handle alone.

When I was a freshman attending the University of Michigan, I was nervous about the things all new college students face their first time away from home, including friends, roommates, schoolwork, and other challenges. Thankfully, my mother, my absolute best friend, was there for me. I'd call her every day, at least once—according to her, it was many, many times a day, but who's counting!—and this was well before cell phones; only a single phone was available in each dorm room to call in or for outgoing collect calls. I'm not sure how I would have dealt with the stresses without being able to confide in her, despite raking up thousands of dollars in long-distance collect calls! Having my mother to talk with made a huge difference during that time.

My worst nightmare since I was a little kid was that my mom would die, and I wouldn't be able to survive without her. In second grade, she told me she'd eaten a cookie that a chipmunk drooled on! (She later told me she'd been bitten by one but didn't tell me because she knew I would worry about her.) I spent the day asking every teacher I could find if you could get rabies from ingesting chipmunk saliva. As a physician, I now know rodents like squirrels and chipmunks do not get or transmit rabies;[10] I wish my elementary school science teachers had known that! My vivid second-grade imagination had me terrified most of that day that instead of getting to a New York City audition, my mom was on a street corner, foaming at the mouth, dying of rabies.

Sadly, many years later, I had to face my fear of losing my mother. Even as an adult with a child of my own, I wasn't sure how I could learn to live without her. We still spoke every day, many times a day. I'm embarrassed to admit that with the advent of cell phones and free long distance (thank you, Verizon), we sometimes even watched TV together on the phone in the evenings; please don't judge me! There were times that I felt like I couldn't even make any decisions without my mother's advice. But she did tell me at one point that her guidance was just about supporting my decisions and giving me the time to realize them for myself.

What I learned from her unconditional love and unwavering support was that she had instilled in me a resilience and strength I didn't realize I had until I needed it. In understanding this, I was able to learn how to bounce back and become an even more resourceful person. I learned how to adapt, survive, even harness it all to become successful.

Losing my mother and having that hole in my life was a difficult lesson I still work through today, but I've learned how to not let it consume me. Surviving that enormous loss taught me how to not only gauge other stresses but also how to manage and cope with them. There are tons of practical ways to cope with stress and be better for it. Coping and managing stress is a lesson that we all need. I'm afraid our next generation is becoming a Prozac nation, being prescribed anti-anxiety and anti-depression medications before targeting the root of their fears and learning simple and powerful coping skills.

When young people today report the typical stress and anxiety, it seems the default move is to put them on medications. Maybe some of them do need that help, but they also need to learn to face their fears, be resilient, and how to cope with life's disappointments and tragedies. These are life skills that we all need to master.

Don't get me wrong, there are certainly times when we need professional help and medical intervention. It is important to recognize the signs and symptoms that you need help. I'll cover that more in chapter 9.

A STRESSFUL NEW ERA

Even before the COVID-19 pandemic, stress and anxiety were becoming more pervasive than in previous decades—especially for our younger generation. Much of it is associated with our access to the internet and social media. While it can be a useful tool to help us create, "connect" with friends and family, share ideas and updates, it has turned into a massive popularity contest with virtually all of us comparing ourselves to celebrities or friends who usually manipulate their photos and post on their best days.

Comparison can make us feel like slackers or losers, or less than, even if these feelings are subconscious. Studies have shown that the increase in depression and even suicidal behaviors in adolescents over that last two decades have coincided with the heavy use of social media.[11]

Our Instagram feeds give us more than updates from our "friends" and "followers." Social media is feeding us a new crop of anxieties, largely based on false perceptions. Other studies have found some social media use can worsen depressive outcomes among adults.[12] People rarely post about the bad things in their lives. They post beautiful pictures, often retouched or edited, to make life appear ever-fabulous. You never really know what's real and what's fabricated.

We end up comparing ourselves with other people's social media feeds, and it can get depressing. It feeds into our fears of not fitting in, being embarrassed, of not being good enough, which in turn creates stress and anxiety before we even walk out the door.

Now let's consider the early COVID-19 pandemic, which put all our lives on pause. A CDC (Centers for Disease Control and Prevention) study showed that the pandemic caused an increase in stress, anxiety, and even substance abuse.[13] Worldwide statistics have shown mental health has been declining steadily since the beginning of the pandemic and has not abated completely as new strains pop up and circulate.

It's no surprise that facing the new norm—shuttering indoors, avoiding others, washing hands routinely, wearing masks, and social-distancing—while hearing report after report about the number of cases and deaths skyrocketing around the world, contributed to anxiety and fears, as well as loneliness and isolation, which worsen those feelings.[14]

Another critical, potentially life-threatening consequence of being in lockdown was women and children becoming victimized by a second, less-talked-about epidemic of domestic violence, which appears to have increased during this time.[15]

As the economy stood still, we all felt the pressure to some degree. Then as Zoom use caught on, we tried to stay connected, but working from home, watching many businesses fold and incomes disappear, we couldn't help wondering if life as we once knew it was over. And sadly, experts still wonder if we are better equipped for the next pandemic—because there will be others.

Another problem we have today is endless media reporting, on TV and social media, highlighting animosity and divisiveness. During the pandemic, it was about public health; now it can be insurrections, elections, instability of world peace—all of this cycling on the news 24/7, contributing to severe mental health consequences.[16] A study published in *Lancet*, and said to be the first worldwide estimate, found anxiety and depression soared by more than 25 percent in 2020, delivering a rippling effect throughout society and homes everywhere.[17] This accounts for an estimated 76.2 million new cases of anxiety brought on by the COVID-19 pandemic alone, with women being the most impacted.

Social media again aggravates this societal stress and anxiety. For many, social media becomes the primary news source, but unfortunately, much of it is unsubstantiated and uninformed. Our X (formerly called Twitter), Facebook, and Instagram feeds spin into another world of conspiracy theories, laced with misinformation masquerading as truth.

Conspiracy theories don't help stress levels. In fact, they enable distrust in authority, which was found to be very dangerous, especially during a public health crisis like this past pandemic.[18] They also can cause people to abandon and distrust anyone with differing views including, loved ones and family members, causing more isolation and disconnection. This creates a vicious cycle, pushing people further down the social media rabbit hole, connecting more and more with other strangers on the internet believing and/or pushing these conspiracy theories. It's clear to me social media's biggest danger is these unchecked "facts" and "theories," which are spreading faster than any virus can.

But it doesn't have to be that way. We don't have to fall for this trap. We don't have to accept and believe every scary idea put out there. We are adults; we must use our heads and be skeptical of things that sound too outrageous or too good to be true, and sometimes listen to our gut when it tells us this can't be happening. We should try not to have an emotional reaction to everything we see and read. Sometimes, we must be less trusting, more critical and questioning, and check the validity of some of our sources.

The other danger of social media is getting caught up in false realities of perfection and beauty, because the media glamorizes perfection. Believe me, I know a little about the perfectionism trap.

PERFECT PEOPLE, PERFECT TRAP

My kindergarten teacher told my mom, "Oh, you're going to have problems with Leigh. She's a perfectionist." As a 5-year-old, I would practice printing my letters over and over until they were perfect. Doing homework as a schoolgirl, if I made one mistake, even at the end of paper, I'd rip it up and start over—because erasing the pencil marks would look too dirty on my sheet of paper! I was always trying to do everything perfectly. When I was really young, before I could tie my own shoes, I would make my mom go back and forth retying the left then the right over and over again until the snugness felt completely equal on both feet. Eventually my mom said, "That's it. We're getting slip-ons!"

To this day, I look at my eyes in pictures and it bugs me that one eye is smaller. I am always thinking about what angle the picture is taken from so I don't notice as much. I know intuitively that nobody has perfectly symmetric features, but that bit of perfectionism in me still drives me a little crazy. When I see myself on TV, I berate myself: "God, that nostril really looks bigger than the other. I should look down more," or, "Boy, that angle really shows one of my eyes is smaller than the other; I should have turned a bit." Crazy, I know, but at least I know it, and I can make fun of myself about it.

My perfectionism has cost me money too. When renovating my guest bathroom, I decided to listen to the sales person who said it would be nice to place the tiles I bought vertically. I wasn't positive what I wanted to do, so I decided to run with the salesperson's idea. The contractor went to work and didn't realize he was working for a perfectionist. When I came home to check out the progress, I saw the wall they finished and said, "Oh my God, I hate that." I had to pay extra to rip it out, buy more tile, start over, and lay the tile the way my gut initially told me to, horizontally.

Sometimes my perfectionism can cost me emotionally too. When my son was in fifth grade, he had an architecture project and was making a model replica of the Mont-Saint-Michel monastery, which essentially takes up the whole island off the coast of Normandy, France. It turned out pretty darn good. Since it's on an island, I could barely contain myself when he didn't finish painting the ocean blue all the way to the end of the board his structure was sitting on; it drove me crazy. When I asked him if he was going to do that before he finished, he said, "Nah, it's good enough."

"Really? Are you sure you don't want to paint it all the way to the end?" I tried to get him to reconsider.

"No, Mom."

"But does it look perfect?"

He turned around and looked at me, "Mom, nothing in life is perfect." I was like, "Oh great, we have a 10-year-old philosopher."

I am ashamed to say that after he went to sleep, I finished painting it blue to the edges. He didn't speak to me the rest of the weekend; he was so mad. Talk about meddling moms, guilty as charged.

However, in the ER, perfectionism is a good trait to have. Well, maybe being meticulous and methodical are better terms for approaching seriously ill patients. As an ER doctor, you don't want to miss anything, and you want to check everything with a fine-tooth comb. Emergency departments are pretty hectic places, so it's critical to have methodical, repetitive procedures to go through when dealing with life-or-death situations, such as trauma codes.

I remember a huge lawsuit in New York City I had read about, where the doctors were called to treat a trauma case: a patient with multiple stab wounds from a fight. When treating trauma patients, we talk about the primary survey, which is the initial assessment to treat imminent life threats.[19] We call it the ABCs, where you evaluate the patient's airway and their breathing and intubate them if needed, then their circulation (for example, if they are in shock from blood loss, we may need to pump in IV fluids).

After that primary survey and stabilization, you must do a meticulous secondary survey, a head-to-toe assessment to identify any other significant injuries that need evaluation and further treatment. In an ER, failing to do a meticulous primary and secondary survey of the trauma patient, which always includes front and back examinations, is a cardinal sin. However, in this New York case, they did not flip the patient over and look at his back. The patient was bleeding into his chest from a posterior stab wound, but they never saw it. He only had a few superficial stab wounds in the front, and they pushed him into a corner, waiting for X-rays and other lab tests, where he eventually died. So, while being a perfectionist in many parts of one's life is challenging, and annoying to loved ones, when it comes to your emergency physicians, most patients would agree it's a good thing.

Being meticulous and methodical isn't reserved for trauma cases. One night in the ER, my neurotic perfectionism paid off again. The patient was in her late 50s; she'd arrived complaining about a painful rash on her pinky finger and was quickly shuffled into the fast-track area where less urgent cases are treated, which is where I was assigned that night.

During the full body survey, I noticed the rash was extending up her arm, in what we call a dermatome pattern along the nerve. Rashes can be due to a wide variety of causes, so I started asking questions while observing her further.

"Ever have chickenpox?" I asked.

"Yes, when I was young," she said, ruling that out.

"How long have you had this rash? When did it start appearing on your arm?"

"Just in the last few days," she said. With her other hand, she started rubbing the middle of her chest and burping. "I've been under a lot of stress lately, and I have this terrible indigestion and nausea too."

"Shingles can come out during stress," I said.

As she went on, I started to suspect something else. She explained that she had been having a very stressful time with her son, and she had been very fatigued.

"You know what? I want to get an EKG and check your heart, OK?"

"If you think that's necessary, sure, but I don't have chest pain," she said.

Within a few minutes, my suspicion was confirmed. She was having a heart attack, and she didn't realize it. Heart attacks present different in men and women,[20] which I discuss further in chapter 8. In men, we see crushing chest pain and shortness of breath. Women, however, often don't have these symptoms. They can just have insidious, nondescript symptoms such as fatigue, nausea, indigestion, sweating, and even changes in sleeping patterns.[21]

If I hadn't been methodical in her survey, this woman who was having a heart attack but complained of a rash could have been sent home with only an antiviral prescription for shingles! I later visited her in the ICU, and she was relieved, and thanked me for being so thorough.

Still, in most cases, we must accept that nothing in life is perfect. In those cases, we are better off just letting go, trusting ourselves to be able to face the consequences, if there are any.

The 19th century poet Robert Browning wrote the poem called "Ixion," a figure from Greek mythology known for his defiance of the gods, which led to a severe punishment. It is frequently referenced in classical literature because it imagines what is possible if we learn from our mistakes. No matter how many times we fail or make bad decisions, Browning implies, we can always find hope, grace, and renewal if we are willing to grow. He stated in the poem, "Out of the wreck, I rise." I learned this during my early days on television, which at the time was harder to break into than getting into medical school. However, through dogged persistence (and almost a few restraining orders) I finally wore down a local TV news director and got my break on WBAL-TV.

Although I was happy to have the opportunity, I started to feel the flutters of anxiety. But I managed my way through the segment. Not long after, I was asked to do a piece on breast cancer in the studio. I remember being nerve-wracked, so I prepared notes for the producer to put on the teleprompter. When it was time to present, my eyes were glued to the screen, and I read my notes aloud verbatim. It sounded so scripted, not at all conversational, and I could tell it was coming out terrible!

I thought, *Oh my God, here I am doing what I've always wanted to do, and I suck at it!* I was stiff and stumbling throughout the segment. During the break, one of the producers came over to me.

"Leigh, you're the doctor. You're the expert. You know more than anybody else here. Don't pretend to be the anchor and read every line perfectly. Just be yourself."

It took me a minute to grasp what she was saying, and she was right. I had to embrace who I was, believe and trust in myself and my expertise, just as if I was talking to a patient, which I do all the time.

Everyone can have anxiety about being on TV. In my case, I realized that I was more anxious about being perfect, which shouldn't have been a surprise. I was trying to cram too much information into a short segment. I just had to make sure I conveyed the key components in easily digestible and understandable sound bites. So I coached myself into believing I was the expert they were interested in hearing from, and to let go of the perfectionism in me. And remember it's okay to "mess up" and make a few gaffes when I'm not in my scrubs. It's something we all do in regular conversation, in fact, it made me more human and relatable.

We all make mistakes, and we all must learn to move on. After realizing this, I began to love sharing my expertise as a medical analyst in the media. And while the emergency room allows me to affect change only one patient at a time, when I speak on TV and radio or write about these issues, I get to affect broader change, impacting health throughout a whole community. As I always said, I worked in the ER to support my broadcasting habits!

Key Takeaways

- Attitude is so important to our mental health. Stress is a reaction to a fear or emotion, which begins with our thoughts.
- Negative emotions and thoughts negatively impact both our physical and mental health. It is important to intervene and address our feelings to put the situation in perspective.
- A conscious decision and effort to be both grateful and empathetic can help release stress.
- We (especially women) must learn how to cut ourselves some slack and not take ourselves too seriously.
- Finding the laughter and seeing the comedy in our own situations can relieve stress. We all make mistakes, but we all must learn to move on from them

Chapter 3

Motherhood Madness

Tick, tock, tick tock ... That was the deafening noise in my head as I felt my biological clock winding down! I thought, as many women do, that I was made to have babies, so when I didn't, I blamed myself. My first marriage didn't last because I was young and consumed with work as a surgery and urology resident. So, after finishing another residency in emergency medicine, in search of a second go-around, I was 35 years old and worried that my chances of having a baby were starting to dwindle. Like many women, I put this added biological clock pressure on myself, not to mention the awkward conversations I pushed about childrearing philosophies on first dates. This had most men running for the hills! And this was without any real personal experience or evidence that I had or would have problems. But in my twisted hypochondriacal mind, each passing day diminished my chances.

I am sure these added pressures also slowly chipped away at my second marriage too. Instead of enjoying our beautiful honeymoon in southern France and Monaco, I made it a baby-making mission. I had convinced myself that if I didn't get pregnant on this honeymoon, it was a sign that my marriage was doomed.

But I did actually get pregnant on our honeymoon and was both relieved and elated. However, at the beginning of my second trimester, I had a miscarriage. I wasn't sure how to read into it. Was it in fact an omen? I insisted on an autopsy with chromosomal evaluation of the *products of conception*, as they are called, after my D&C (dilation and curettage)—which is the standard of care and routine after miscarriages. They did find a chromosomal abnormality that was incompatible for sustaining life. However, this only further confirmed my deepest fears that my eggs were just too old!

For the next several years, we tried, unsuccessfully, to conceive. We then started the fertility clinic treadmill, as I called it: weekly doctor's appointments for diagnostic workups and therapeutic treatment. Despite not finding definite organic physiological reasons with either my husband's or my apparatus, the doctors agreed that due to my "advanced maternal age," we needed to go straight to the in-vitro fertilization (IVF) route. I started a regimen of injecting myself twice a day, while my husband's biggest challenge was navigating traffic while driving 100 mph to get his fresh sperm to the clinic on time.

The fact that I could not get pregnant after the miscarriage was driving me crazy, as I felt my biological clock was ticking away. The more I worried, the more stressed I felt, and we know that stress has negative effects on fertility.[1] This just sets up a viscous cycle. Studies have shown that infertile women who are taught behavioral stress management and relaxation techniques not only had measurable decreases in their psychological distress, but also had increased their conception rate.[2]

However, that is easier said than done! Two years passed, and the whole process was nerve-wracking. I just wanted a baby, but my body was not cooperating. Women often feel like such failures when something that nature has designed perfectly just does not seem to work, and I was no exception. I also had a complication from the IVF called ovarian hyperstimulation syndrome[3]—a condition that occurs when the ovaries blow up to the size of a grapefruit, from overstimulation from all the IVF drug treatments. You tend to gain weight from internal fluid build-up everywhere, which besides making you look like the Michelin Man can also be dangerous. It causes abdominal pain, nausea, and vomiting, as well as potentially fluid in your lungs.

They wanted to hospitalize me. Infertility was consuming my whole life. On top of this, my husband was petrified at the thought of having multiple births, which is common with the IVF procedure. Although we were able to produce plenty of embryos, we only inserted a few at a time, which further lowered our probability of getting pregnant.

After several dreary and very expensive cycles, we decided to give up, take some time off, and regroup. I canceled the rest of our appointments, and I went back to focusing on my career. In a strange sense, it was a relief. Now I just had to focus on doing what I loved and let the marriage run its course while we considered our next option. But a funny thing happened. A few months later, I did get pregnant—naturally.

In my last trimester, I was giving a talk at a hospital where my fertility doctor worked. Looking at my baby bump, she asked, "What happened to you?"

Well, you could have called when I canceled all the rest of my appointments to see what was going on, if you really cared, I thought. *I only spent almost every week with you the last several years!* But instead, I said, "I told you I did not have a physical reason for my infertility." As soon as I canceled our appointments, and stopped all the treatment, my body finally said yes.

I know stress caused the prior failures. The stress hormone cortisol did a number on my life, obviously. But as soon as I let go of my plans to get pregnant, my body said *It's time!*—which can happen more often than people realize. You often hear of women who, right after they adopt, become pregnant. While it is hard to find data on this phenomenon, an older study from 1963 found that around 10 percent conceived after adoption.[4] And they stated it is probably in women without documented physical abnormalities causing the infertility.

While some fertility experts may dispute this, despite not actually adopting yet, just by stopping the stressful IVF cycles of trying, for me, it was true. Other studies have shown that about 20 percent of women who needed fertility treatments, such as IVF, to conceive their first child are actually likely to get pregnant naturally in the future.[5]

You would think that having such a rocky start with getting pregnant was one of the most stressful things that I had experienced, but unfortunately my pregnancy was no picnic either. My first trimester, I had hyperemesis gravidarium, a condition of intractable vomiting.[6] I spent that time either face down in the toilet bowl or in bed. Luckily, since my husband and I were both doctors, he brought home IV fluids, so I did not need to be hospitalized. But I lost almost 10 pounds that first trimester. And it was a good thing. I gained over 30 or 40 pounds during the pregnancy. I can imagine how big I could have gotten! I wasn't the glowing, beautiful pregnant woman like celebrities on Instagram. I had zits, hemorrhoids, and was burping constantly with indigestion. A true joy to be around.

In my eighth month, I developed preterm labor and was put on bed rest. I remember visiting my doctor and asking, "What the hell is this big mass near my diaphragm?" I wondered because she had told me she felt the baby's head in my pelvis, and I knew I did not have twins!

"Well, I don't know," she said, which was not very reassuring. "Let's do an ultrasound to see what's going on."

It did not take long to spot another potential complication of this pregnancy. My baby was breech, meaning his feet were down and his head was up, pressing against my diaphragm—hence the horrible reflux and burping. What she was feeling in my pelvis was a huge fibroid preventing my baby from turning head down that would probably obstruct his exit.

Considering my age and these conditions, she said, "You know what? I think we should do a C-section."

Not wanting him to get too much bigger, we scheduled for surgery within a couple of days. The day arrived, and I elected spinal anesthesia, which caused nausea and retching from lowering my blood pressure. But my baby boy arrived. When the doctor lifted my baby out to show me, despite being covered in blood, my laser-focused eye saw a bleeding, vertical laceration on his butt.

"He's cut. That's a laceration! He's cut," I yelled.

The doctor said, "Yes, I know. I'm having a plastic surgeon come in to look at it. I'm so sorry."

The plastic surgeon came in and said, "I think he'll survive this." Now, I haven't seen my son's butt for many years now, so I'm assuming it turned out okay, but thank God he was breech. Otherwise she could have cut his face, while struggling with my fibroids.

I had so many fibroids that she was having a hard time putting my uterus back together. Later, she told my mom I almost ended up with a hysterectomy and that I would probably have a lot more complications with the next pregnancy, which subsequently never happened.

WORRY WARRIOR

If you think infertility, pregnancy, and birth can be stressful, actual motherhood brings a whole new batch of stresses, and in my case, dare I say, madness. As a first-time mother, I brought Max home feeling like I was in a boat without a paddle. Indeed, there are no training manuals that fully prepare a new mom for what's ahead, including the stress of caring for a newborn.

It's like trying to protect a helpless life from every imaginable danger. Moms become worry warriors, whether we want to or not. And as an ER doctor who has seen the worst, I was sure dangers and disasters lurked at every corner of our home.

Everyone knows that sleep becomes more valuable than gold those first few months. Like many new moms, I seemed to sleep with one eye open for the first few weeks. Then, wouldn't you know it, his colic suddenly started right at the textbook time: at 2 weeks old.[7] It was like clockwork. At the stroke of 6 p.m., the colic cry-storm started and then ended at midnight.

I'd strap him to my body and do everything around the house in the evenings with him attached. He would scream the second I put him down and even when I tried to just sit down. This pre-dated the Fitbit and Apple watch, but I must have clocked over 1,000 miles those months!

During that time, my husband had a golf weekend planned. I panicked and pleaded, "Don't go. Please, don't leave me with him; please don't go."

"Sorry, this is what I planned," he said as he walked out the door.

At the end of my rope, completely exhausted and overwhelmed, I called in the cavalry in the form of a baby nurse. She was fabulous, and it turned out to be the most relaxing weekend I can remember in my life. I slept, which was heaven on earth. I then cleaned out my closets, which always relieves my stress. I was able to get some other things done, and I started feeling human again.

When my husband got home, the nurse was going to leave, and I pleaded again this time with her, "Please don't' go!" Looking at my husband, I said, "Maybe you should go on another trip."

NIPPLE SAVANT

My mother didn't breastfeed me as a baby, which was normal at that time; not many mothers did. There was pressure to use pharmaceutically created infant formulas. This was also probably encouraged by my physician father who worked in the pharmaceutical industry, which falsely boasted that new formulas promised to have more nutrition than breast milk.[8]

By the time I became a mother, the science had caught up and mother's milk was reaffirmed as superior. I felt enormous pressure to breastfeed, or risk my son being malnourished, having less immunity,[9] and worse—not getting good SAT scores, as many reports at the time were claiming. The pendulum had swung the other way, and studies were coming out declaring higher IQ in breastfed babies.[10] When pumping my breast milk into bottles, I feared he would have the dreaded "nipple confusion" that breastfeeding advocates warned about, the idea that he might not be able to go back and forth between the breast and the bottle. I was consumed with fears that he would not get into a good college, and it would be all my fault!

I was set on breastfeeding, but during the first week of having Max at home, I was really struggling with getting him to latch on. With my hormones raging, being overly tired, not feeling well, and crying from my perceived rejection and feelings of guilt over not being a good mother, I asked a La Leche nurse—part of a breastfeeding crusader movement called the La Leche League International—to visit me to help save me from this lactation stress. I remember showing the nurse my nipple and crying while I asked, "Is it going to fall off?" It had a three-quarter inch circumferential ulcer on it and appeared to be hanging by a thin thread of tissue. Plus, I had a bad case of mastitis, an inflammation and sometimes an infection of the breast tissue.[11]

"Oh God," she gasped. "That looks terrible. I don't think you should breastfeed like that. You know it's bad when the La Leche nurse says, "Oh, dear. I would go to the bottle right now."

"Are you sure?" I asked, fearing my son's mental and physical development were at stake.

"Oh yes, that's the worst case I've ever seen," she said matter-of-factly. But she reassured me he would be okay and that I needed to cut myself some slack. I thought to myself, *We'll just have to make up the breast milk deficit with an SAT tutor!*

Good thing he turned out to be a "nipple savant." He was a genius at transferring back and forth between the bottle, the breast, and even the pacifier (something that I thought should surely be included in his college essays!). I was able to use a breast pump and feed him breast milk from the bottle. But after a while he graduated to formula.

You'd think that as a doctor I'd be able to make precise calculations when it came to making the formula, but I didn't realize the damn 8 oz. Playtex bottles with plastic liners are really only 5 fluid oz. and that I needed fewer scoops of formula powder. I was giving him a concentrated formula, plumping him up very quickly.

My mom noticed it too, "Oh, no wonder he loves the formula now over your frozen breast milk [which was thinner]. It's like a formula milkshake!"—which is why he rejected all my frozen breast milk at the end. So that's an important fact to take note of for moms using those those bottles, and I feel they should have a warning label for sleep-deprived mothers!

I wrote the following article when my son was already a teenager, but back when he was little, I was nervous about pacifiers too.

Pacifier Relief for Mom in Time for Mother's Day
A new study brings great news for us guilt-ridden moms who used pacifiers to calm our kids.

By Leigh Vinocur, MD
A new study[12] brings great news for us guilt-ridden moms who used pacifiers to calm our kids.

It's been 15 years for me, but I still remember the dilemma when I took my newborn baby home from the hospital: To suck or not to suck? As a working mom, I was well aware of the binkie controversy. At first it seems cruel to me, giving my baby something to suck that provided no sustenance. But he took right to it, and I soon realized that the sucking instinct in newborns goes beyond feeding. In fact, babies in the womb can be seen sucking their thumbs on ultrasounds. This phenomenon is called non-nutritive sucking,[13] and it even exists in animals. So why have pacifiers been given such a bad rap? Many hardcore breast-feeding-only moms harbor the long-held belief that using a pacifier or artificial nipples will interfere with breast-feeding. They theorize that this can cause the dreaded "nipple confusion." They argue that pacifiers can inhibit your baby's ability to learn to latch and suck properly, as well as possibly decrease the duration of breast-feeding.

Well, there is finally some prospective research data to back up us pacifierists, as I like to call myself! Pacifierists are the weary working mothers just looking for a little bit of peace (and quiet). Some of you may not be aware of the shame and agony we have had to endure at the hands of the breast-feeding advocates when we gave our babies "pacies" to calm them down.

The new, small study out of Oregon Health and Science University[14] shows that this notion of pacifiers interfering and preventing good breast-feeding may not be the case at all. Researchers looked at 2,250 infants born between June 2010 and August 2011 and found that when pacifiers were only allowed for limited, supervised use by nurses and not routinely available for moms, there was not an increase in breast-feeding, as they had expected.

In fact, the opposite occurred. They found a significant drop in the rate of breast-feeding after pacifier restriction, from about 80 percent to 68 percent. In addition, after restriction of pacifiers, researchers also found an 18 percent increase in—I dare not say, but yes—formula use! Despite this encouraging study, many staunch breast-feeding advocates are still not convinced.

In my own experience as a mother who succumbed to the allure of the "binkie," I found that my son was apparently some form of nipple savant. He certainly didn't have any nipple confusion. In fact, he was able to use and discern between those nipples on my breasts, those on a baby bottle, those used by the sitter with my pumped breast milk and even the ones on the pacifiers! Yes, he could use them all and go back and forth in between them hourly with ease, he was ambi-nippleous!

As a physician and a mom, I am well aware of the benefits and the importance of breast-feeding. The list of benefits is endless. In the past, physicians spoke of its importance in bonding and passing your immunity on to your baby. However, recent research goes beyond that. There are studies that show it can decrease the risk of childhood obesity, and for heaven's sake, some studies even tout higher SAT scores (well at least higher IQ!). While advocates stress the longer the better, if your kid can ask for some milk to put in his coffee, I think enough is enough!

I don't intend to diminish in any way the importance of breast-feeding. However, I often feel too much pressure is put on new moms. I am against hard-core extremists that guilt you into doing it longer or more often than you are comfortable doing. I remember my own experience with a horrible infection and nipple ulcer—I thought my nipple might fall off, but I was determined to continue to feed and pump. And to this day, I still have this irrational fear that if my son does not get into his first choice of college, I know I will still blame myself for quitting too early!

Hopefully, this new research can start to put to rest the pacifier guilt and will stop hospitals from locking down the binkies as if they are controlled substances!

And for those addled, sleep-deprived moms whose kids continue to shriek, even after they have been breast-fed, rocked, walked, vacuumed near them for hours, placed on the washing machine or in the car circling the block for the 100th time... enough is enough... just stick a pacifier in his mouth.

If only it was that easy to quiet a surly teenager!

Originally Published on HuffingtonPost.com

There are also other issues related to pacifiers and thumb sucking, like dental problems, such as preventing teeth from coming all the way down if used too long, but I had a pediatric dentist who told me, "Look, pacifiers are better than thumbs because you can take them away, but in either case we can always fix his teeth; you can't fix his personality if he needs a binkie to soothe at night."

And that little binkie made my son and me happy. Of course, I know there's no real scientific correlations between pacifiers, personalities, and how far your child will go in life. Often, we find our kids survive and thrive despite our parenting decisions and skills.

Sometimes we get so mired down in the rearing of our children and the worrying about their future that we miss the fun and beauty of the present while they are growing up. My mother, who always looked on the sunny side and lived in the moment, often reminded me of that. She loved my son to death, calling him, "The Bard of Owings Mills." He was the Shakespeare of our town. He did sometimes say the craziest things; she even started journal with his various phrases she called "Maxisms."

One time, as a three-year-old from his high-chair, he picked a cherry up by the stem and spoke to it with a love sonnet. "Oh, gentle cherry, loyal servant to my tongue."

Another time, also as a toddler, he opened the window in the backseat of the car and said, "I love the taste of the wind in autumn," then he opened his mouth and took a gulp of fresh air. I guess it's no surprise that he went on to college to study both physics and creative writing.

When it came to my son's health, it seemed everything I learned in med school went right out the window! As a worry warrior, I was always second-guessing myself.

As far as I'm concerned, there is no such thing as a stupid question, especially if you are a new mom! Somehow, to my surprise, by the time my son made it to the ripe old age of 10, I only had to change pediatricians twice. The fact that I've never had him opened for exploratory surgery for a tummy ache is a testament to the medical profession, and the sanity of his father.

Never mind that I made it all the way through medical school and residency with good grades and board scores. In fact, as a cavalier resident rotating through pediatrics, I used to roll my eyes when hysterical moms brought their kids into the ER at 1 a.m. for the sniffles. But once I became a mom myself, I totally understood it. When I first looked at that little face smiling up at me, knowing I had waited so long for him and tried so hard to have him, my rational, analytical medical brain turned to mush.

Maybe it's my training as an ER doc that teaches me to think of the worst-case scenarios that can happen in an emergency to treat them. But when treating patients, I can turn it off and become the sensible, level-headed physician

I need to be. I'm actually very calm and collected in the ER, even under the direst of circumstances. In my residency training, I worked at a trauma hospital for children. I saw the most horrific cases of children paralyzed from motor vehicle accidents, gunshot wounds, and cancers. I was cool as a cucumber.

My first job out of residency, at a small community hospital, I saw a child who fell into an open dishwasher and was impaled through the neck with a steak knife. I calmly secured the child's airway, put her on a ventilator, stopped the bleeding, and arranged for transport to a pediatric trauma center. I did all this while calming the mother and the child, who incidentally after repair of her esophagus at the other hospital, did fine and was eventually discharged home. You can bet that I never allowed any knives or forks to point up in my dishwasher after that!

So why doesn't this calm turn on with my own son? When he was tired and upset, instead of concluding that he could just have a headache, I'd jump to thoughts of a brain tumor. I'm not alone in this. It's a mother-doctor thing, because one of my closest friends from medical school was convinced her tiny infant swallowed the nipple part of a pacifier that had broken off when she couldn't find it. She took her child to the ER, which resulted in an endoscopic exam using a lit tube with a camera down the child's stomach to look inside. Of course, the nipple wasn't there! Obviously, this is the very reason doctors should never treat themselves or family members.

At least, I can now hand that hysterical mom in the ER at 1 a.m. a tissue while I hold her hand and emphatically say, "I totally understand."

BABYPROOF EXPERT

People used to joke that I could go into someone's house, point out every potential hazard and danger, and babyproof it from top to bottom. In fact, I even did a segment on WBAL-TV where I told people to get down on their hands and knees and crawl around their house to find all the potentially dangerous things that kids could get into. During the taping at my house, I gave my then toddler a "child-proof" pill bottle for demonstration. While I was on camera telling viewers to make sure all their meds are in baby-proof bottles, my little Houdini somehow managed to pop open the bottle.

While trying not to crack up on-air, I had to pivot the conversation to say this was a demonstration that there is "no such things as child-proof—only child-resistant" and that "there's no replacement for being vigilant." You've got to love live television.

As my son grew up, it's safe to say I was extremely cautious. I imagined just about every possible way he could be killed or maimed so I could reverse-engineer a way to prevent that from happening. The combination of the perfectionist ER doc inside me and the professional worrier made me a little compulsive about his safety. If I could have wrapped him in sanitized bubble wrap, I would have.

I joke about the stress of parenting for me, but I know I was lucky to have a high-paying career, and despite getting divorced when my son was young, I was able to afford help. For many women, especially those who go it alone and must work several jobs just to makes ends meet, stress can lead to serious physical and mental health issues.

Studies have shown that greater levels of parenting stress are associated with poorer physical health, lower quality of life, and psychological health.[15] Additionally, while there has been some jest in the idea of chardonnay-sippy cup moms and mommy-wine culture, there are dangers in making light of this.[16] Studies have found that women are catching up to men in the incidence of substance use as a coping mechanism.[17] It is important for women to address these issues and the stressors causing them, as well as to seek professional mental health support help as needed.

It is critical to have a support system as well as to make time for yourself. For me, it was my mother who provided the support. Thankfully, my son loved spending time with Nana and Popi Edi at their home in Lake Placid. It was great for all of us. We made memories boating on the lake, skiing, playing games, and enjoying the quaint town. There's nothing like handing off your little one to Nana!

If you think your young children can be stressful, those teenage years can also be very difficult—especially their final year of high school. In fact, some studies have found that during this time, there is enough stress in parenting to turn to alcohol.[18] For parents, it can feel like this is when the rubber meets the road. Often, we feel it is the ultimate test of how well we raised our kids. Teenagers today put a lot of pressure on themselves as well—based on social media and societal expectations to go to college, which I admit is not for everyone. It's hard to separate yourself from your kids as they try to navigate their way through young adulthood and inevitably face disappointments as they try to figure what is next for them.

It makes us think back on own lives, our choices, and how they affected our self-esteem and self-worth. I know for me that self-doubt was real, but I always had my mom to talk with, and she always had a way of making me feel better. But now as mother, I realize that perhaps her unburdening me might have caused her to internalize my worries, since I know that is how I feel about my son. I don't know who said it, but it is so true: "You're only as happy as your most unhappy child."

But I do know I am lucky to have a somewhat similar relationship with my son; he knows I'm always available for him. Although boys are very different, when he calls, he does not really want my advice! For a perfection- ist ER doctor mom who feels she has to fix everything, it can be really dif- ficult to bite my tongue. But he just wants me to listen to his complaints or his venting while I try to calm him down and make him feel better.

That's what's funny about raising kids. They go from being snugly babies who rely on you for everything and think everything you do is the best, to suddenly thinking nothing you do is right and that you don't know anything. But I think I might have done something right. He's working on a PhD, has a great sense of humor, and still stays in touch with me.

It's funny, my son had a surrogate grandmother who was a close family friend that we both adored; she never married or had children, and I always joked that's why she lived to age 98! The point of this chapter is to validate for you that these stresses we feel as mothers are real! When we feel con- flicted in loving and hating our kids at the same time, science backs us up; the jury is still out about whether motherhood is good for us!

Telomeres are the end caps in our DNA that protect our chromosomes from essentially fraying when our cells divide.[19] They shorten with aging, dis- eases, and stress and their shorter length has implications related to a shorter lifespan.[20] Some studies[21] report that pregnancy and childbirth shorten our telomeres and accelerate aging, while others suggest that motherhood slows down our aging.[22] There are even some studies that state that women who become moms when older, like myself, may actually have longer telomeres length.[23]

Despite the stresses, I am still glad I became a mom. But I do want to talk about a serious topic related to mom stress: postpartum depression.[24] While it is true that hormone shifts, physiological changes in your body, along with lack of sleep and worries about being a good mom can affect your mood and cause the "baby blues," it is important not to minimize these feeling, espe- cially if they get worse. Studies have shown that there is an increase in the incidence with up to 20 percent of women experiencing serious depression after giving birth.[25] This puts moms and their babies' health at risk, as well as increasing the risk of suicide for these mothers.[26] A recent study found the number of new moms killing themselves within the first year of childbirth has tripled this last decade.[27]

It's important to remember, like with any type of serious depression, this is a chemical imbalance that needs treatment, not a personality fault. If you have feelings of hopelessness and intrusive thoughts of harming yourself or your baby, *do not* feel ashamed. Let your family and healthcare provider know immediately so that you can get treatment. There is even a new, faster-acting anti-depressant[28] on the market now to specifically treat postpartum depres- sion, so do not suffer in silence!

FROM MOM TO MOI

If you have made it to this stage in life with your kids out of the house, congratulations! But now, as I like to say, it's time to go from Mom to *moi*, the French word for *me*. Meaning, it's me-time! Time to regain your physical and mental health after the kids have flown the coop. You are done with the mad dash after work as well as running around on weekends to sporting events, theater, music, and dance recitals. You survived the stress of the SATs, ACTs, the AP classes, the college applications and visits. Even though your kids were such pains in the ass those last few years when you dreamed of shipping them off, you managed to get over the surprising sadness and trauma of actually dropping them off at school.

So, you ask, what now? Well, I found there are a plethora of books, articles, as well as segments on morning news shows on how to cope with being a new mom and what to expect, but there is a void on the topic of being an old mom!

It's like getting a second life, a time to pursue your passions and take back your sense of self. It's a great opportunity to reinvent yourself. It may sound scary or stressful, and may cause some anxiety about the challenges ahead, but I'm here to tell you, empty nesters have the opportunity to rise up and begin to reach for their dreams and aspirations. After all, we've come through one of the most difficult experiences in life—having and raising kids!

Later chapters will help you embrace these changes and navigate the new stresses and anxieties ahead. As long as we are alive, we really can't avoid these, but we can learn to manage them and thrive. So cut yourself some slack about what you might have done better during those years of child-rearing and focus your attention on what will make you happy now.

Key Takeaways

- Raising kids is hard and an imperfect science with both great and horrible times for every mom.
- There is no such thing as the perfect mother, so cut yourself some slack
- If you rely on alcohol or substances to relieve your parental stress, it's important to ask for help and support.
- If you are having intrusive thoughts about hurting yourself and/or your baby, don't be ashamed. Talk to your doctor immediately as post-partum depression is a serious medical problem that can be treated.
- Once your children are out of your house, it's time to go from "Mom to Moi," taking me-time to find your health and happiness.

Chapter 4

Career Reinventions

Beyond motherhood's maddening stresses, we women share a number of other anxiety-producing opportunities when it comes to our lives and careers. We must endure many stressors unique to our sex that we may not always have the power or control to change.

Today's #MeToo movement has certainly awakened society to the prevalence of sexual harassment. We must supercharge our motivations when facing bullying, income disparities, and finding a voice in the boy's club. We have opportunities to pursue our passions, earn a living, and contribute to society from our vocation. But women have to learn to harness their stress or risk being washed away in the imminent waves of gender-oriented biases and discriminations. Here are a few examples from my own career path.

My professional journey began very early. I believe our career paths begin with the center of any child's life—their mothers. My Jewish mother thought I walked on water and gave me the confidence to believe I could try and succeed at anything!

I remember reading the Amy Chua book, *Battle Hymn of the Tiger Mom*, that caused an uproar. She was criticized for expecting too much of her kids. I remember thinking, *Really? These Chinese moms don't have anything on Jewish moms. We invented the (Saber-Tooth) Tiger of Moms, but maybe with a little less sternness!*

My mom instilled in me the idea that I can do anything I put my mind to if I work hard at it and am willing to try and learn new things. That's why I've had various reinventions on my professional journey—and it is not over yet! Albert Einstein said, "Intellectual growth should commence at birth and cease only at death." I believe that and enjoy learning new things regardless of my age.

People who know me know that my mom was more than my mother; she was my best friend and confidante. It was her unconditional love and support, with no harsh pressure, that propelled me to take chances and risk putting myself out there to try anything new that interested me and not be afraid of failure. Her support allowed me to reinvent myself and my career many times over.

That's not to say we agreed on everything. She let me make my own mistakes, and I have certainly had failures along the way in life, love, and marriage. Growing up, when in school, I wasn't the best standardized-test taker but still got all A's in high school. When my admissions counselor told me I was admitted to the University of Michigan Honors Program and said she thought I would excel in college but didn't think I should go into medicine because of all the standardized testing, I said to myself, *Really? Just watch me.*

I am one of those people who never takes no for an answer—whether I am ordering off a menu, returning a purchased item, or trying to get a new job. I'd rather take charge of situations than let things linger in limbo. When you combine these traits with perfectionism, perhaps my mother created a monster, but at least a productive one.

One summer, I came home from college unhappy. Despite not having any experience, I talked my way into working at a local restaurant. This gave me the perfect opportunity to focus on something other than school and to make some money over the summer.

Within a few weeks of working as a waitress, I was promoted to daytime manager and had my first experience of work stress. I remember reversing some numbers (and letters; I probably had a bit of dyslexia before it became a thing) on the accounts, and spending hours going over every digit until I found the error to close out the books every day.

One day, only the cook and I showed up for the busy lunch rush. Sure enough, that was the day my parents decided to come visit me at work. Despite having no hostess, no waitresses, and no bussers, I swallowed the stress and put it to work.

I settled into an extreme focus. As the guests came in, I helped them find a table, took their drink orders, then went and made their drinks (often cocktails. I took their food orders and placed them with the cook. Then, I handled the next guest and the next. The cook was flipping steaks from his grill in the dining room area, and I was scooting around from table to table, from the back kitchen to the tables, like I was on roller skates. It became quite a spectacle.

Soon, every table in the restaurant was filled up, and I was taking care of everything but cooking the steaks. I was all over the place, making drinks and appetizers, slinging plates, pouring water, taking the checks, picking up dishes, and then onto the next guest—all with a smile on my face. At one point, the cook just stopped to watch.

"I can't believe you're doing this," he said, watching me multitask like an octopus juggling act. Once the first rush finished and all the tables were dirty, I just threw bus pans on the floor in between all the tables and started chucking in dirty dishes (luckily none broke); I pushed them all into the back kitchen and then started again with the later lunch rush. Rinse and repeat!

At one point, the guests actually started applauding me. Sometimes it can be surprising finding your resilience and rising to the occasion in a stressful situation. This certainly portended my choice to go into emergency medicine, since it has a similar pattern of running around and multitasking!

The next day, the restaurant owner heard what the cook and I accomplished. "Want to be the full-time manager and run the whole restaurant?" he asked.

I talked it over with my mom. Although my parents caught the show, they didn't want my career to be in the food service business. "Are you kidding? You're going back to college," my mom said. That was the extent of my restaurant career. I guess I retired at the top of my game!

MOVING INTO MEDICINE'S MALE WORLD

I love learning, so moving into medicine was a good choice for my professional journey because there's plenty to learn. In many ways, those days at the restaurant and other summer jobs all helped lay a foundation for my medical career. I'm always growing, learning, and juggling caseloads to help others. So, after earning a Bachelor of Science in biology at Michigan, I went on to obtain a Doctor of Medicine at Wayne State University. During this time, I realized I would be a woman in a male-dominated field; I'd have to sink or swim with the boy's club. At the time my medical school class had less than 30 percent women. Today, many have equal numbers of men and women, and some skew with more women in their class.[1]

It didn't take long to be harassed. In my second year in medical school— which was before the #MeToo movement—I was in a class learning about physical diagnosis and listening to the heart. We had a male family practice doctor who was either volunteering or on faculty, who separated the men and women and gathered the women into a room.

"OK, now you're going to practice auscultating and percussing on each other," he said. With auscultation we use a stethoscope to listen to heart and lung sounds, and a slight thumping on areas of the chest called percussing to listen for different resonating sounds.

He continued, "Now, I want everyone to take their shirts off to help with the exercise."

As a few participants started unbuttoning their shirts, my lab partner leaned over to me and said, "I'm wearing a high-waisted girdle; I am embarrassed to do this."

"You're not taking your shirt off!" I told her, then looked at the doctor and said, "Are you kidding me? We're not taking our shirts off. We are more than capable of completing the exercise with our shirts on."

Later, I complained to the dean, and I believe there was some kind of disciplinary action taken. But this kind of thing happened all the time.

I started my medical career with a residency in urology, which is unusual because there were hardly any women going into this field 30 years ago. When I applied less than 1 percent of urology residents were women.[2] But I loved the challenge. I was into the feminist ideal that came from Helen Reddy's feminist anthem album called *I Am Woman.* I was traveling all over interviewing for different urology programs and at one, after a series of all-day interviews with various faculty members, which I thought went very well, my last was with the chairman of the department.

After I walked in, he motioned for me to shut the door and sit in a chair across from his desk, then came around and perched himself on the edge of his desk and said in a rather low voice, "I just want you to know that I'm never going to have a woman in my urology program. I just invited you here to see if your ass looked as good as your face" (we had to send a headshot with our applications). Startled, stunned, and eventually pissed since this was not one of my top choices anyway, I stood back up and looked him in the eye.

"Really, asshole? This may well be the last time you see it!" I said, and turned around and walked out, slamming the door hard.

A UROLOGY EULOGY

My top choice was my program at WSU because they had one of the top pediatric urology programs in the country. My idol and mentor was one of the top pediatric urologists in the country. His name—Dr. Alan Perlmutter—a key author on the cover of the main textbook, *Campbell's Urology.* I had been doing research with him in medical school and he was the one who encouraged me to go into urology and was appalled by what had happened. When I was accepted at WSU, I became the first woman ever accepted into their urology residency program. But I was also the last woman they would have for at least 10 years after I left toward the end of my fourth year before finishing. I still feel bad about that.

Being a pioneering woman in urology brought about its own set of stressors; I'd be the butt of crude jokes and my fair share of sexist and misogynistic remarks, which even started during my first two years of surgical training, required before I could even start my three years of urologic surgical training.

During one surgical rotation, I decided to get a perm because always wearing a surgical cap over my hair, after hours of surgery, my hair would be flat as a pancake. I thought it was easier because I could just wash and go.

After one long session in surgery, I pulled my cap off and *poof!* My hair popped out. One of my surgical attendings on faculty at the program said, "Hey, Vinocur, where did you get your new hairdo, the poodle palace?"

Everyone laughed. And while I don't think he really intended to be mean, these kinds of comments and awkward situations would never have occurred if I were a male resident. I laughed it off at the time, but always being the butt of jokes was taxing. Another one of my surgical attendings, who was rather old, used to call me "little girl." I know he meant it to be endearing, but it wasn't. And it was unprofessional in front of patients, who already thought I was a young nurse in training. This moniker certainly did not instill confidence in my patients about my capabilities as a surgical resident.

Even though I loved my urology department chairman, Dr. Pierce, my mentor, Dr. Perlmutter, and many attendings, such as Dr. Smith, who were very kind and caring, they did not really understand the stresses of being a woman in the field because they'd never had a female resident before.

I have to say I was rather sheltered at the time. I grew up in a household where my mother never said *vagina* or *penis.* She'd just call both a "front tushy!" I remember my first rotation was at the VA hospital; I was working with Dr. Smith and going into my first patient's room ever in urology to evaluate them.

"Good morning, Mr. Jones" I said cheerily. "What seems to be the problem?"

"It's my Johnson," he said.

"Oh, I am so sorry, Mr. Johnson," I replied. "I must be in the wrong room. I have Mr. Jones's chart."

"I am Mr. Jones," he said.

"But you said you are Mr. Johnson?" I asked, confused.

"No, it's *my* johnson. My peter," he retorted.

"I am sorry, I don't understand. Who exactly are you? Are you saying you are Peter Johnson, not Thomas Jones?" I replied again.

This went back and forth for a while, when I heard my attending hysterically laughing outside the door. He came into the room and explained that vernacular that I had never heard of until that day. Still laughing, he wrote out a glossary for me on slang words for male genitalia so I could finish my clinic day in time. That was eye-opening for me. Johnson, peter, snake, tool, and rod were names for penis; nature, seeds, and rocks all equaled testicles.

There were other challenges too. I remember one night I was finishing up and had to track down one of my chief residents for sign-out rounds. I found myself in an awkward situation when he insisted that I come to him, but he was in the male doctor's locker room to do it. I was thankful most of them were in towels.

This was a time before the "little blue pill" arrived to treat men with erectile dysfunction, so I had an andrology clinic where we worked up men for evaluation of implanting a penile prosthesis. As part of the workup, I spent nights up in the sleep lab setting up strain gauges on their penises to watch them during sleep to see if they had night-time erections. I would have to bring in husbands and wives to discuss masturbation techniques as well as show them how to use a device called a vacuum erection device.[3] They are actually still around and now have a battery pump, but in the old days, I would have to show the couple how to slide a tube over the penis and pump out air manually to create a vacuum, which then pulled blood into the penis to make it more rigid. After that, a rubber band was pulled down to the base of the shaft to hold the blood there for a semi-rigid erection. If all this failed, they would be put on the schedule for a surgical penile implant.

It was strange that once people knew I was a urology resident, friends, family, and even strangers would ask me their most intimate questions for advice. Once, I was sitting at a restaurant for dinner with a very close friend and her parents. Suddenly her mom asked, "You know, Leigh, every time Jerry ejaculates, nothing comes out. Why is that?"

My dearest friend shrieked, "Oh my God, Mom, this is not the place!"

Needless to say, Jerry looked very uncomfortable, embarrassed, and pale too!

Over time, all of this was taking its toll, my first marriage was crumbling, and I began to question my career choice. I entered the program because I knew ultimately, I wanted to be a pediatric urologist and do a fellowship at Children's Hospital of Michigan with my research mentor, Dr. Perlmutter. But urology was an early match, so I didn't actually do my pediatric urologic rotation until my fourth year of medical school, after I had already matched at WSU department of urology. It was ultimately a traumatic experience that made me think perhaps I should not be in the residency. Residency placement, even back then, is facilitated by a computer that matches you to a program based on your ranked choices and the program's ranked choices.

During that rotation as a fourth-year medical student, I was scrubbed in on a surgery (just holding retractors) with a 10-year-old being operated on for a massive cancerous tumor in his abdomen called a neuroblastoma,[4] which already had a bad prognosis for its size and someone his age. When one of the residents removed this tumor, the size of a volleyball, it must have torn a major blood vessel. I watched blood fill up this child's whole abdominal cavity and spill over the sides to the floor. He coded—his heart stopped—instantly and a cardiothoracic team was called in and spent the next 10 hours trying to close the torn vessel and revive him with blood transfusions and cracking his chest for open cardiac shocks and massage.

I stood there the whole time holding the retractors, not moving a muscle. The room was so quiet except for the instructions called out by the surgeons. The team stopped heroic measures around 10 p.m. and "called the code," as we say, pronouncing him dead at that time.

The surgery had started at 8 a.m. and I was exhausted so I went to sleep in the doctors' OR lounge. When my hero and mentor, Dr. Perlmutter, came in and sat down next to me, he was devastated and visibly shaking. He quietly sobbed about losing a young boy on the operating table, mumbling about even having done this operation thousands of times, getting so cavalier that you don't order the angiograms anymore, which would have outlined the blood vessels better to pick an approach for removal.

He surmised the tumor was fed off a blood vessel directly attached to the largest blood vessel in our body—the aorta—and that's why he bled out. He was the country's top and most respected pediatric urologist, and if this could have happened to him, I thought to myself, *I can't do this.* I couldn't live with myself if it happened to me. In the ER, while you do face life-or-death situations, patients come in already in dire situations that are not of your doing.

I felt like I tried urology, which is a very narrowly focused specialty, and my interests had always been broader. After all, I studied history in college along with molecular biology. And I couldn't imagine the emotional toll of pediatrics.

So I left near the end of my fourth year of urology training even though I only had one year to go before finishing the urology program. To this day people ask me, "Are you crazy? So close to finishing?" But you must be true to yourself. It probably would have been easier to just finish. Despite it all, I actually did well in that residency; therefore the agonizing decision to leave was very hard to make. I felt like I was letting everyone down: my chairman, my attendings, and my fellow residents, as well as womankind—being the first at WSU! But it was the right decision for me.

You must believe in yourself. I took a big leap and pivoted relatively late in my residency career. Many of my friends who did internal medicine finished by year three and were looking for jobs or fellowships, while I was about to start over in a new field of medicine. And this was just the beginning of me challenging myself to keep moving and learning new things throughout my life. Being ready to fail is part of the learning process.

Of course, my mom told me that she was happy about the decision, even though I had spent all that time only to figure out it wasn't for me. She always told people I was a neurologist, not urologist, anyway, because she couldn't stand me constantly using the *P* word—penis—in conversations!

FITTING INTO THE ER

Once I left urology, the surgery program asked me to come back and finish general surgery residency. I thought about doing that and possibly getting into plastics, which would have been another three years of general surgery and three more of plastic surgery, which probably would have been the best thing for me to do because I'm very good with my hands, and I could have made a fortune. But I was exhausted with all the education, so I took six months off to think things through.

During that time, I decided to start working in a walk-in clinic at a nearby hospital and cover for a nursing home practice family doctor. I started to see that emergency medicine was a better fit. Plus, the ER gave me lots of flexibility to explore other non-medical opportunities.

Emergency medicine requires a broader-base medical knowledge. It was exciting to me. I felt like I could actually make a difference treating people, working as a team trying to turn terrible situations into positive outcomes. There's nothing wrong with helping older men pee or get erections; it's a noble cause, but just not for me at the time. Plus, I've always felt the ER represents a microcosm of society.

As an ER doctor, I treated all the medical problems and social ills we see in modern life: problems related to obesity, smoking, teen pregnancy, drug abuse, mental illness, gun violence, and domestic violence. I saw this abuse seemingly every day. In one pivotal case, I learned early on that domestic violence (DV) knows no socioeconomic boundaries—and you *cannot* pick out those at risk.

I remember an 80-year-old woman who kept returning with injuries from "falls." The doctors kept working her up for mini-strokes and seizures, as the causes. But when I saw her for the first time with my astute senior resident, we finally asked her if someone was doing this to her. "Yes," she said, her husband of 60 years.

No one, including her own doctor, had ever thought to ask. After that, I knew that I would screen everyone with this line of questioning. According to the National Coalition Against Domestic Violence (NCADV),[5] one out of four women will experience intimate partner violence in their lifetime. It was then that I committed myself to working for these women. I began training physicians and worked on a state pilot program in Maryland that led to screening everyone coming into the ER for domestic violence and working with great community programs such as Maryland Network Against Domestic Violence (mnadv.org) and CHANA (https://chanabaltimore.org/), a faith-based domestic violence program in the Baltimore community serving victims of abuse in the Baltimore area.

While I loved working in the ER, I sometimes found it upsetting. Emergency medicine is not preventive health. There were victims of trauma, heart attacks, and advanced cancer coming in during their health crisis and *after* their condition had spiraled out of control. While this was a teachable moment, and I would try to spend some time discussing preventive measures with them; unfortunately, often it was too late. Added to that, there was not a lot of time in a busy ER to spend talking to patients.

My disillusionment with this specialty came when my chairman told me my patient satisfactions scores were off the chart great, but that I was spending too much time talking to my patients, and that I need to move faster! The adage in the ER is "treat 'em and street 'em." Patients were considered relative value units (RVU)[6] and how many RVUs you moved through on your shift determined some of your compensation. While it also assesses the complexity of the medical care documented and administered to the patients, the concept just never sat right with me.

It seemed like there was never enough time to spend with patients, and I would always feel defeated and stressed out by the end of my shift. It is no surprise that according to an American Medical Association (AMA) report, the specialty of emergency medicine has the highest burnout rate at 62 percent.[7] I wanted to find a way to educate and hopefully help prevent their emergency from happening in the first place!

BROADCASTING PREVENTION

This ER experience tapped something inside me—to do more. I've always loved to educate and had some journalism classes and training in school. So I set my sights on medical broadcasting. As opposed to treating and educating one patient at a time in the ER, I could use my medical knowledge to educate a whole community of patients, at once.

Medical broadcasting and emergency medicine are actually more similar than different. In both disciplines you must be ready to handle any situation, any patient or any late-breaking news that comes through the door or across your desk. Both require you to think on your feet. Emergency medicine is the perfect specialty for medical broadcasting because I have to take care of all different types of medical patients, so I am comfortable discussing any type of medical topic. This has served me well on live TV and live talk radio.

Both have inspired me to serve others, now on the front- and back-end of health. I looked at my adjunct broadcast career as my personal public health initiative to proactively help people manage their health and wellness before an emergency occurs. I used to tell people I worked in the ER to support my broadcasting habit, because much of it was pro-bono!

Despite my passion, it wasn't easy to break into television. I shared the story earlier about the determination it took when I mentioned it was easier to get into med school than to get on TV! But finally, I got a job at WBAL-TV as their medical journalist. I also answered questions and shared my insights on health on their radio station. Then, this side career started getting national attention and I started doing segments for national cable news FNC, CNN, MSNBC, CNBC, even *The Dr. Oz Show*. I began my own internet radio show on RadioMD, which was picked up by iHeart radio's new talk platform.

Before my break into TV, I had to accept rejection after rejection, but I actually found it motivating. Just as the Pulitzer Prize-winning poet Sylvia Plath who was often attributed to saying, "I love my rejection slips, it shows me I tried," me too!

I pressed on, determined to help people prevent illness and disease before they wind up in the ER. Since then, I've written extensively as a columnist/contributor for *GreenState*, *Huffington Post*, *Savvy Auntie*, and contributing to the Dr. Oz website. I love writing about important medical topics and tempering the sensationalism in medical news. How often have you metaphorically picked up the morning paper to find another new medical study that contradicts the one you heard about yesterday? I call it the "Study Du-Jour Syndrome."

We live in this information age where complex medical studies are explained in 30-second sound bites. As a physician and a medical journalist, I feel the responsibility to sort through all the conflicting data and weigh in on what's truly a significant finding that has a bearing on someone's health and explain it in understandable English.

I would like to think my work in the media has helped to reduce some stressors for people and given them better insights on related health matters. And, most importantly, helped them avoid crisis situations landing them in the ER!

THE CORPORATE MEDICINE HANGOVER

Some of the most stressful times in my career came while serving as chief medical director for fifteen urgent care clinics. While my heart was in a good place, the corporate culture of medicine in large health systems tended to strangle my efforts to improve the quality of care, just to preserve the bottom line. I wasn't prepared for this kind of work in med school—or to fight workplace bullying. Being a woman in that leadership role is often a battle.

While the majority of medical school classes are now about 53.8 percent[8] women, there's still a huge discrepancy in academia, with only 11 percent of female faculty making it to full professor.[9] As far as leadership positions in healthcare overall, women account for only 18 percent of hospital CEOs, and 16 percent of all deans and department chairs.[10] Women still seem to have glass ceilings and/or sticky floors when it comes to moving up the ladder.

In my case, I helped the business increase revenues by 35 percent, created and oversaw patient quality and safety-risk reduction programs, and improved patient satisfaction. These were all measurable and sustainable, yet I continued to be criticized by the men in leadership roles. Once, I took a phone call at 6 a.m. only to have a male counterpart unprofessionally shout at me about something inconsequential he'd advocated for that I did not agree with. He only backed down when I said I would not tolerate his bullying.

I had to battle tooth and nail to preserve my reputation but also to continue delivering the best care possible at these clinics. This is the kind of stress that keeps you up at night. Many of these situations were out of my control, and I felt vulnerable to imminent attacks.

One day, I thought I'd try discuss my situation with the Chief operating officer, who was a woman. I offered to take her out for coffee, but she never returned my email. It was apparent that I was on my own, which I assumed she'd had to do to reach her position. But I really try to spend my career bringing other women up to succeed with me.

Inevitably, corporate medicine always seems to back the men in leadership more than women. Nobody seemed to care about workplace bullying, including the human resources department. I saw that HR just cared about protecting the company, not its people. I was miserable fighting the system. Incidentally, I was so touched and proud when I left that leadership position in the urgent care chain and several of the women, physicians, and nurse practitioners that I'd hired let me know that they quit when I left! Others that stayed for a bit and then left still keep in touch with me and complain about the toxic workplace environment there.

Toxic workplaces with bullying not only add to your stress levels, but we also know they are detrimental to your mental health. Sometimes it is to the point of requiring medication for anxiety and depression. A study published in the *British Medical Journal* conducted by Finnish researchers found that 20 percent of women and 12.5 percent of men experience workplace bullying, requiring medications such as antidepressants, sleeping pills, and anti-anxiety sedatives.[11] And the bullying that creates such a toxic atmosphere at work is even harmful to employees just witnessing the bullying, who also have a 1.5 times increased risk of requiring medication too!

We know that workplace stress contributes to poor physical health and increased risk of cardiovascular disease. In some studies, there is up to a 40 percent increased risk of heart attack or stroke from workplace stressors.[12] Studies find people harboring anger and negative emotions are more likely to develop premature heart disease and have a greater chance of having a heart attack.[13,14] Funny, how my wise mother's advice resonated true and always put things in perspective for me. I now often ask myself what she used to say to me, "Leigh, is this worth having a heart attack or getting cancer over?"

It was time to let this go and make another pivot in my career. It didn't take long to find something that ended up making me much happier. I started consulting with a firm that genuinely needs my input and appreciates what I have to say.

I've had a great journey during my career, despite the difficulties of breaking into a male-dominated vocation. I'll always be grateful for my mother, who encouraged me to rise in the face of challenges, as well as showing me when it was time to move on. I've stood my ground, made a few pivots, and kept my head high. Ironically, being a woman has some advantages too. In the next chapter, I'll share the little secret that has given me an edge over my male counterparts.

Key Takeaways

- As far as your career, being a woman in a man's world is a constant uphill battle. You need to stand up for yourself because no one else will.
- If a situation occurs at work or school and it doesn't feel right to you, don't go along with it; talk to someone who can help you mitigate it.
- Don't tolerate a toxic workplace environment; it can jeopardize both your mental and physical health.
- Change is hard and presents some challenges; it involves learning new skills and sometimes failing, but that is all a part of living and growing.

Chapter 5

Vanity's Little Secret to a Long and Good-Looking Life

As of this writing, I'm a medical director for a wellness company, a chief medical officer at a nutraceutical manufacturer, I have a small medical cannabis consulting practice, I'm active as a television medical analyst, and a guest columnist for national publications. I spent the last several years caring and scheduling orthopedic surgeries and appointments for my father, who was staying at my home that whole time. I also was caring for a beloved surrogate grandmother with dementia who recently passed away.

My son started a PhD program in graduate school in a small midwestern town during the COVID-19 pandemic. Without any new student activities or orientation, he was thrown into teaching classes virtually and doing lab work all by himself—without guidance from his advisor or even contact with other grad students. It was a stressful time for both of us. Because as I have stated before as in the adage, "You are only as happy as your most unhappy child." I tried to be his support system, but offering advice about a PhD program in physics was well beyond my capabilities—and he let me know that!

At the time, I was also caring for my beloved labradoodle who had cancer and sadly passed away this year. She was a light of my life; I refer to as my "doghter." She was the reason I did not take a real vacation for over fourteen years. As I constantly told my husband, Europe will always be there, but she won't. I have no regrets spending every minute with her while we had her! I always say I couldn't love her more if I gave birth to her myself—and she came without all the stress and drama that kids sometimes bring! But all these stressors, which everyone has in varying forms, compelled me to write this book. Many people have told me they think I have it all together and that I am successfully just breezing through my life. But it is not true! I am no different than you.

Do I have any spare time? Not really, but I do have plenty of stress. I can't tell you how many times I've put off my own doctor's appointments for tests like mammograms and colonoscopies. It is a sad case of doctor heal thyself.

However pathetic as it may be, what I did make time for was my Botox and fillers. You see, my theory when I was younger was to never take a medication or have a procedure unless it had some cosmetic effect. I can see a bit of that fallacy as I am aging now, but I do believe even at an older age that when you feel that you look good, you do actually feel good. And we know how our feelings can impact both our mental and physical health. It is part of my trademarked "Health from the Outside IN.™" There are studies that show appearing older than your actual age is actually a prognostic indicator for poorer physical health.[1] I submit to you that there is absolutely nothing wrong with the desire to look terrific no matter your age.

Today in the US, according to the Centers for Disease Control and Prevention (CDC), 60 percent of Americans are living with at least one chronic disease, like heart disease and stroke, cancer, or diabetes.[2] I believe that vanity is a potential and very powerful asset, one that hasn't been fully exploited to help us stay healthy. When we look good, we feel good, and stress levels decrease. That is why I think vanity has a bad rap. It's defined as, "something worthless, trivial or pointless," but the little secret is we all have a bit of vanity, or the cosmetic surgery and cosmetic dermatologic procedure industry wouldn't be raking in over $82 billion a year. So I say, why not use it to your advantage?

It's like I tell some of my patients, "If you won't exercise for your heart, at least do it for your butt and thighs!" This may seem tongue-in-cheek, but there are virtues of vanity that are advantageous to your health. We women are smart. Of course, we know the importance of being healthy, but what we really want is to look good too, which in turn makes us feel good! There are plenty of medical books on the market today touting the benefits of good health and how to stay that way. Well, as a woman I say that's not enough. I think we are overlooking the primary motivator that will get us to do almost anything if it serves our appearance.

I always tell my own doctors, "My low blood pressure is really just the collateral damage of my lean protein, lower carb, high omega-3 diet intended to keep my tummy flat!" Let's face it; aging is no fun. As a doctor and medical broadcaster, I'm always touting health advice, but it's really the sheer terror of my dropping boobs and expanding waistline that keep me off a lot of rice, pasta, and bread.

What I've found is that pure vanity fuels my drive to stay healthy. I still believe I can have your doctor applauding your triglyceride levels, which are really a result of slimming your belly and thighs! When I speak publicly, I always get asked how I stay fit. When I mention my age, people seem surprised. So why not reveal my secret? Unlike these coming-of-age beauty books, with their flowery clichés about aging gracefully with total acceptance, honey, as far as aging, I am not going quietly!

I believe in not aging gracefully, and I am reluctantly going kicking and screaming the whole way! In fact, it's this insane urge that gets me out of bed in the morning to hit the spinning bike and treadmill. Or spend oodles of cash on the latest wrinkle creams and minor procedures. This is also why I don't go in the sun without being completely covered up and slathered with SPF 50–100.

I am grateful for both my medical career, which allows me to make a difference in the life of one patient at a time, and my medical broadcasting career, which allows me to make a difference in the lives of the broader community. Taking your health seriously can also mean taking your beauty seriously; they are, in fact, related. There is nothing wrong with cosmetic procedures to create your best-looking you, but there has to be a healthy balance as well. We should practice moderation.

Our celebrity-crazed nation is fixated on looks and appearance. It's estimated that over 15 million cosmetic procedures are performed each year in the US.[3] Despite the pandemic, a study in 2020 found that Americans still spent $16.7 billion on aesthetic treatments and cosmetic surgery.[4] And so many people travel to other countries to have procedures that there's a name for it: medical tourism.[5] When people seek out surgery to change something about their appearance, they often have a specific celebrity in mind. They ask for a nose like Scarlett Johansson's, Jessica Alba's, or Ashley Simpson's. Kim Kardashian and Selma Hayek top the list for butts, while Jessica Biel and Liv Tyler have the most sought-after lips.

This is actually a red flag.[6] As we discussed prior, you should just worry about your best looks rather than constantly obsessing and comparing yourself to other people—especially celebrities, who have teams of people to make sure they look good, and only show their best faces on social media. The obsessing and comparing is detrimental to your mental health. The obsession with one's perceived physical flaws is called *body dysmorphic disorder* and is especially common in teenagers and young adults.[7] Social media has been magnifying this, causing body image dissatisfaction, depression, and eating disorders.[8]

While I submit to you that there is absolutely nothing wrong with the desire to look terrific no matter what stage you're in, it must be tempered. I submit to you that there is a dichotomy and apparent disconnect between our quest for beauty and the miserable state of our health. More than half of all Americans have at least one chronic disease,[9] with obesity now classified as a chronic disease and one of the major contributors to others like heart disease, diabetes, high blood pressure, high cholesterol, liver disease, sleep apnea, and certain cancers. Therefore, I have always seen the potential of using our vanity as a powerful asset; it's one that hasn't been fully exploited. Perhaps it can become your motivation to make those healthy lifestyle changes.

Health happens to be one of the most important and magnificent "side effects" of paying attention to your appearance because well-being and beauty are intrinsically intertwined. When we look good, we feel good, and that can decrease our stress levels. Why not use what really motivates us —vanity—to make serious shifts in behavior that will leave us looking our sexiest and most appealing at any age? We just need to take care of ourselves on both the outside and inside.

HEALTHY BEAUTY, HEALTHY BODY

This shift in thinking certainly helps me. As a physician and a televised medical broadcaster and national columnist, I'm always on top of the latest research and health advice. I know from seeing patients in my practice as an emergency physician that poor health and lifestyle choices have a profoundly negative affect on quality of life. But I have to admit to myself, and to you, that I sometimes practice what I preach out of the sheer terror of not being able to fit into my jeans. Vanity keeps me healthy. And I know I too must learn how to temper this!

For example, I can laugh at my vanity. After coming through my cardiac stress test with flying colors, my friend and cardiologist told me that because of my family history, he might consider prescribing a cholesterol medication called statins if my blood test results were outside of the normal range. When faced with the possibility of needing a pill, I thought to myself, *No way. I don't want to be on a script for the rest of my life, unless it could have a positive cosmetic effect!* Then I thought about it a little longer and realized that having uncontrolled levels of cholesterol and triglycerides *could* also wreak havoc on my appearance.

Xanthomas, small or large (some bigger than 3 inches in diameter!) yellow bumps of fat, are common in people with high blood lipids, and can pop up on lower eyelids, elbows, joints, tendons, knees, hands, feet, and even on the tush. Crap! Yellow fat bumps on my face and ass? You've got to be kidding. No way I'm going there. So, if I do need them some day, I will bite the bullet and take a statin. I have taken a prescription for acne and ointment to smooth the occasional eczema patch, not to mention my daily drops of Latisse, a prescription that helps my eyelashes grow long and lush, so what's a little statin to keep my lower lids and rear end smooth?

Believe me, I don't love passing up a warm, crusty baguette or dragging myself out of bed to exercise. I certainly wouldn't do either one just to make my lipid panel look beautiful. Exercise keeps my heart pumping, but it can also make my stomach look flatter in that little black dress. In fact, waist circumference measurement is actually a parameter that cardiologists now use to assess risk for heart disease. Studies show excess belly fat, aside from causing that muffin top on your jeans, does lead to increased risk of heart attack, diabetes, and stroke.[10]

Exercise is also critical to maintaining our muscle mass. After age 30, you can lose up to 8 percent of your muscle mass per decade, and even more after the age of 60. Reduced lean muscle mass not only leads to serious mobility issues later in life leading to disability. It also makes your thighs look like cottage cheese due to cellulite, for which inactivity is one of the risk factors,[11] and who needs that? And maintaining your lean muscle mass also raises your resting metabolic rate, so you burn more calories at rest.[12]

That is why my vanity approach works on patients too. Women who have not yet started to see the effects of their decisions on the aging process are sometimes hard to convince with the argument to do it because "it's good for your health." When I tell these women about diet and exercise, or medicines that can help them control cholesterol and blood pressure (I'm all for pharmaceutical intervention when necessary), I get rolling eyes or sighs in return.

But when I tell them, "Okay, if you won't do it for your heart, do it for your face and your hips." *That* message seems to get their attention and they see healthful practices in a new light. In fact, this type of reasoning also works for teens. A study showed that anti-smoking advertising campaigns seemed to fail when just health messaging was used as opposed to tying smoking directly to its negative effects on attractiveness.[13]

THE MIRROR FACTOR

My nana had the old-fashioned view that vanity was a crime against modesty and humility. She thought that gazing in the mirror posed a risk; we could become dangerously vain. That was a dirty four-letter word for her! However, I disagree. As a recovering mirror addict, there is nothing sinful about looking in that mirror and learning to love yourself. It can be a useful tool! And I have written about it before.

Confessions of a Mirror Addict
By Leigh Vinocur, MD

I am writing in defense of the mirror! A *Today Show* segment highlighting Autumn Whitefield-Madrano's blog on HuffPost[14] on "mirror fasting" struck me as odd. More than odd, actually—it is a form of denial, the proverbial ostrich sticking its head in the sand! Don't pay attention or don't look and it doesn't exist.

I can still hear my Nana's voice: "Leigh, stopping looking in the mirror, it will make you vain!" She had those old-fashioned views. Every summer as a little girl when I came from New York to Michigan to stay with her, the first thing she did was change my cool 70s hippie middle hair part off to the side and throw out my black dresses and shirts. "Little girls shouldn't wear black, it brings bad luck."

As if just by looking at yourself in the mirror you could become vain! In fact, to her vain was a four-letter word. She was from the hearty stock, a working woman back in the 40s while my mother was little. The original Rosie the Riveter, she had no time for frivolities. Although I never really believed that, because why would she bother with her full-length girdle if that was the case!

Nevertheless, she instilled enough guilt in me that it took me quite a while even with the unconditional, supportive love of my mother to be happy with myself and love myself. And that journey did begin with my mirror!

So, all this talk of mirror fasting echoes of Nana Irene, but I feel it is sending the wrong message to young girls. Because we can't blot out all reflections of ourselves, or we will have to cover up completely. We need to use the mirror as a tool that reflects and allows us self-reflection.

We need to let women know it is only their reflection they need to be concerned about! Don't look into anyone else's mirror. There shouldn't be any comparisons to magazines or runways. We need to stop the quest for "the" ideal of beauty and find our own ideal of beauty, both inside and out. Look into your mirror and pick out one thing you love about yourself and start your reflective journey into self-affirmation! We need the mirror as a tool to instill confidence in young women. A Glamour magazine poll[15] found that 97 percent of women have a negative body image, with on average 13 negative body thoughts a day about themselves. That's about one an hour when we are awake! Ladies, we are in some serious need of self-loving, and it all can begin in the mirror.

As women, we put ourselves last behind everyone—friends, family, sometimes even our pets! We are the caregivers to all, and often this selflessness can be to the detriment of our health. I have seen many women patients in the ER who run themselves ragged from being pulled in so many different directions. For years they have not taken care of themselves both outside and in, and now they are reaping what they have sown in the form of a stroke or heart attack. In fact, often they even argue with me that they don't have time to be admitted!

By looking into our mirror and saying that we love ourselves, we can begin the journey. You need to say to yourself you are worth the effort. The pride you take in yourself and your appearance says you care about yourself, and it is reflective of your health. There is science behind the "bad hair" day.[16] If we look good, then we tend to feel good about ourselves, and that, in turn, can translate into health.

My premise of health from the outside-in is that the things I do to help enhance my appearance to stay thin and fit, such as exercising and eating healthily, also obviously positively impact my health.[17] From my own experience, I find the days I run around doing everyone's else errands without time for myself, in my sweats with dirty hair pulled back, are usually the days I self-indulge in junk food and have a harder time motivating myself to work out. And as a celebrity-crazed nation with an obesity epidemic, we obviously aren't heeding the message we doctors give about beautiful, pristine arteries, so why not focus on the outside if people will listen to that? Then the inside will fall into place.

Of course, as a physician and a woman, I am cognizant of not becoming obsessed with my looks. But really, who among us multitasking working moms even has the time for obsessing about that? I am giving you permission to take some time for yourself. Spend a little time primping and pampering. Vanity is a virtue when it comes to your health and if the journey begins with your mirror, so be it!

Originally Published on HuffPost.com

I know that an obsession with appearance can have harmful side effects; we've seen the images of women who take plastic surgery and crash-dieting too far. There is such a thing as an addiction to cosmetic surgery.[18] And we know that there is such a thing as making ourselves sick from an obsession with being thin; it's a condition called anorexia nervosa.[19] Both are symptoms of deeper psychological issues associated with body dysmorphia. Studies in the scientific literature have found a correlation between body image distortion and poor mental and physical health outcomes.[20] These instances are indeed concerning, but prevalence of an actual diagnosis of these conditions are still less common than what most of us suffer from, which is a lack of healthy self-esteem.

Most of us are in some serious need of self-love. In fact, the mirror can be a valuable tool that can help instill confidence as I said previously. We need to look in that mirror and give ourselves the gift of self-acceptance. And it can start by identifying just one feature that we like about ourselves, and building on that affirmation every time we take that morning glance in the mirror.

Over 40 percent of the US population is now suffering from obesity,[21] and about 43 percent of us are dealing with a chronic disease due to our poor lifestyle choices.[22] Physicians are failing in our messages to patients. Either patients don't listen to us or what we tell them doesn't resonate. I think it is the latter. When I tell a patient that she should exercise or eat well or stop smoking or overdoing the saturated fats and simple carbs because it will make her *look* so much better, I get a different reaction from the typical glazed-over look that comes when I start talking about LDL and HDL numbers. Premature aging is also primarily the result of lifestyle choices too.

Of course, much of this is tongue-in-cheek to a degree, because too much vanity does have a ridiculous side. Much of my adult life is a good example of this. I am not ashamed to admit I have been known to go to extremes that I have to pull myself back from. For those of you who have already bought into my premise, I'm sure you have your own examples of the absurd lengths that we go to in the name of vanity. Thanks to my mother, I have a sense of humor about myself, and that is important for your health too. Occasionally, I must check myself and say, *Leigh, the mirror is the beginning of the journey, not the final destination.*

Healthy vanity is an active form of balanced self-esteem. The opposite can be extreme humility in the form of "letting yourself go," which can be bad for both your looks and your health. Women who don't value their appearance at all often don't value other aspects of themselves. Research finds that low self-esteem often manifests itself as personal neglect,[23] and that's dangerous for both your mental and physical health. When feelings of low self-esteem are accompanied by worry and anxiety, they are also followed by high blood pressure, depression, and stress, not to mention the associated wrinkles and obesity.

Women with a healthy sense of self tend to take better care of their appearance, but that can translate in to taking better care of your physical health, too. Studies have found that improving self-care and confidence lead to significant improvements in a patient's ability to follow through with medical treatments, which in turn help them manage their chronic medical conditions, as well as help them maintain important lifestyle changes even during times of stress.[24]

In essence, if these patients need to be treated for these conditions, on average they *recover faster* than those who don't. A researcher from the University College in London published a study that found that those who experience more joy and optimism daily have a positive picture about themselves and their self-esteem, that this optimism biologically keeps them in a relaxed, non-stressed state that enables these thoughts to thrive.[25] People that are optimistic with a positive mindset also have lower levels of cortisol, a stress hormone resulting in better health.[26] This study looked at over 200,000 people and found a 35 percent lower risk of developing cardiovascular disease such as heart attack and stroke, as well as a 14 percent lower risk of early death when compared to pessimistic people. They also have better results following surgery and fewer complications and have better coping skills.

A healthy dose of optimism and self-esteem contribute to better sleep,[27] which is a factor in coping and handling stress. Therefore, by accepting your healthy dose of vanity, I believe, as corroborated by research, that your stress levels will decrease. I'm not suggesting you need to keep up with the Kardashians, or anyone else for that matter. Just stay beautiful according to your own beauty standards. And beauty is more than skin deep.

The only person you need to appeal to is yourself. The trap of trying to look like a celebrity is not the point. But tapping into vanity's dirty little secret can motivate you to care for yourself and, ultimately, make you feel better. It goes beyond self-esteem to the point of self-compassion,[28] being kind to yourself, forgiving yourself, and understanding and accepting your imperfections because *no one* is perfect. And this is what this book is really all about.

Key Takeaways

- VAIN is not a dirty four-letter word!
- Vanity gets a bad rap; a healthy dose of vanity can bolster your self-esteem.
- Make self-esteem and vanity about self-acceptance and loving yourself.
- Spend time looking in the mirror to find at least one thing you love about yourself to start your self-affirmation journey.
- No one is perfect; accept and embrace your imperfections.
- It important to have self-compassion and be kind to yourself. Don't compare yourself to anyone else's notion of beauty, only your own.

Part II

HOW TO HARNESS
STRESS FOR SUCCESS

Chapter 6

Tips to Harness Stress

As you may have gathered by this point, I've handled and harnessed as much stress as anyone, despite people thinking I have it all together! I tear out my hair, figuratively, worrying about an array of issues and, I deal with as much stress as everybody else. I have overcompensated for it, leaned on my mom, faced my fears, focused on the task at hand, called for help, reflected, learned from it, laughed it off, pivoted my career, applied my vanity, and when none of that works, I scream into a pillow, just like you!

Along the way, I've learned there are good and bad ways of handling stress. I know we're all different, but we're also a lot alike. As I said, we all have stress because that's how our body works. I know that stress and anxiety can get out of hand and require professional help. God knows, I've gone there. There's absolutely no shame in having a therapist. In some cities, like New York, it is an essential accessory! Through my journey, I've found several ways to calm myself down, which are backed by science and research. Here are my Dos for harnessing stress. And my Don'ts are coming in the next chapter!

FIND A FEMALE DOCTOR

It's not because I am one. Sorry, gentlemen, female doctors just seem to be better. That is, if you're measuring patients' longevity. A study found you're more likely to live longer if you have a female doctor.[1] Researchers published findings from a four-year study in the *Journal of the American Medical Association* (JAMA) measuring patient outcomes, comparing the results with male and female doctors. They found that patients treated by female doctors had lower mortality and less hospital readmission rates than those cared for by male doctors. The study suggests there are differences in how male and female doctors serve their patients. They found women doctors are more likely to practice using approved clinical guidelines, while also ensuring their patients are engaged in preventive care. And we are better listeners and communicators,[2] taking the time to listen and engage in positive talk and psychosocial support.

The same goes for when you're going under the knife. A recent study in *JAMA Surgery* [3] found that female surgeons have lower rates of postoperative complications, hospital readmission rates and bad outcomes, including death, at 90 days and one year after surgery, when compared with those treated by male surgeons.

From my experience, I make sure I take the time to listen and understand my patients. I'm more of a quality-oriented than quantity-oriented doctor. I know there are plenty of great male doctors out there, but there's nothing like a woman doctor who genuinely cares, who is both patient and thorough.

In the past, the medical profession was dominated by men. The days of women being treated for being "hysterical" for just about anything and prescribed valium by male doctors are over. In fact, today female physicians account[4] for over one-third of the US physician workforce and comprise half of all US medical school graduates. Unfortunately, there's still quite a disparity in academic leadership positions, as well as leadership positions in the medical corporate world, with less than 20 percent being women.[5] Therefore, if you're looking to harness stress and live longer, find yourself a woman to be your doctor.

Use Your Smile's Secret Weapon

How you look and express a positive outlook is just as important to success as being intelligent. When I was in my 20s, I would walk the University of Michigan campus looking sour and miserable, perhaps because of typical coed insecurity or the belief that my seriousness was I indicative of my intellect and young adult angst. Of course, it could have also been the gloomy Ann Arbor winters, but that is something we will discuss later. Often, I looked so glum that people would ask me if there was something wrong, which only made matters worse!

Later, when I was in my emergency medicine residency, I had an epiphany in a bar with a girlfriend. We had a bet: Could we get any guy to come over and talk to us? So, I looked around, picked the best-looking guy in the bar, made eye contact, smiled at him, and what do you know? He came over and talked to me—and ended up asking me out!

That was a powerful moment. I realized then that you could use your smile as a secret weapon. Who knew it could be that easy? Flexing a few facial muscles was easier and less risky than a wet T-shirt contest. And I felt empowered when I overcame my fear of rejection; I felt happier, sexier, and more attractive. As I've gotten older, I have learned to lean into engaging others with eye contact and a warm smile. A study[6] revealed that both sexes found the opposite sex more attractive and approachable if they were making eye contact and smiling.

The converse is also true;[7] studies have found that overusing the muscles in the face that cause frowning, even if you initially feel happy, can make you feel sad and depressed. Interestingly, a study out of University of Cardiff in Wales[8] found that treating patients' frown lines with Botox injections, which paralyzes the muscle movement needed to frown, can make people feel happier with less negative emotions[9] than those who could make a frown. And the same researcher also found, in another study, that using Botox on laugh lines (such as crow's feet) [10] was associated with higher depression scores.

So aside from not overdoing your Botox injections so that you can, in fact, still smile, this also underscores how our emotions and feeling are tied to our facial appearance. I know it can be hard to paint on a smile when going through tough times, but the point here is to try to check your attitude because we've already learned how harmful negative emotions are for our health. Additionally, in these recent times of political stress and divisiveness, when you disagree with someone, and you can calmly debate them with a smile (and facts), it's actually much more disarming! Plus, attitudes are contagious; True smiling can make us more beautiful inside and out. And we should be using this secret weapon to our advantage!

Be Your Own Cheerleader

As we've learned, stress and anxiety are linked to our fears, and perhaps a feeling of being ill-equipped or inadequate somehow. We can't let our fears end up defining who we think we are! We must develop a kind, compassionate, and positive attitude toward ourselves as we discussed in the last chapter. Low self-esteem is a world-wide problem. It's estimated that 85 percent of the population[11] has low self-esteem.

Research shows[12] that low self-esteem is dangerous for both your mental and physical health. Feelings of low self-esteem can be associated with poor health behaviors, such as alcohol and drug abuse, smoking, overeating, or poor eating and exercise habits. All of this can lead to anxiety, depression, obesity, heart disease, and diabetes. Even people who might have a predisposition for a disease like diabetes and heart disease from their family history may *never* get the disease if they take care of themselves as a part of maintaining their good self-esteem. And if they do need to be treated for these conditions, people who believe in themselves *recover faster* than those who don't.

A study[13] reviewing many research articles on the topic showed that those with higher self-esteem and emotional well-being not only recover faster from physical illness, but also have better long-term prognoses with those illnesses. A University College in London study[14] showed that those who experienced more joy and optimism daily had a positive self-image and had overall better biological function. They had the lowest levels of cortisol, the hormone related to stress and hypertension. The participants also had better heart rates and blood pressure and had a much lower risk for a heart attack than those who were pessimistic and without joy.

Forget the Holy Grail quest for *the* perfect body and focus instead on achieving *your* perfect body. Learn acceptance and compassion without compromising your standards. For instance, my legs are never going to be longer than they are. That's unfortunate, but it's also reality. I'm not going to let that stand in the way of my cultivating a great attitude and taking care of myself. I can do everything possible to make my legs look longer, such as wearing high heels, but optical illusions aside, I'm just not going to give my legs the power to determine how I feel about myself.

While it sounds cliché, you've got to believe in yourself and be compassionate, too. Like Henry Ford said, "Whether you think you can or think you can't—you're right." So, you must think you can! There is truth in the power of positive thinking.[15] Taking control of your thoughts can help you control your emotions. A smart friend and psychologist colleague once told me, "As you think, so you shall be."

Therefore, find something that reminds you that you are valuable and uniquely wonderful. Identify any shame that has defined how you think about yourself and forgive yourself. If you are lucky, you may find that special person in your life who reminds you that you are loved regardless of your bad hair days. But remember, you don't always need someone else to do that. Get yourself a new hairdo or new outfit or total makeover to boost your self-esteem and be your own cheerleader!

Learn to Forgive for Your Heart's Sake

Holding onto, obsessing over, and ruminating on resentments and grudges hurts you more than you may realize. Harboring this resentment and feeling of being wronged can foster feeling of unforgiveness that can be the root of stress and anxiety. Often this unforgiveness hurts us much more than it hurts those who we feel have crossed us. It is toxic. And while I'm not telling you to be a doormat and let people walk all over you, recognize that everyone has their own set of problems and can act out in unfortunate ways. Whether you feel like you might have a played role in the situation or that you didn't and are being wronged, taking some responsibility for your actions and feelings thereafter can be helpful in finding room for forgiveness.

Besides, forgiveness does your heart good. Think about those situations in which you feel someone, or something is unfair to you, and it makes you angry. Notice how your heart begins to pump faster. Studies done on healthy students just imagining someone or a situation where they were angered, wronged, taken advantage of, or hurt caused their heart rates to jump almost two beats every four seconds above baseline. When they held a grudge, it rose almost three beats and increased their blood pressure over 2.5 mm/Hg.[16] Over time this takes a toll on your heart.

What ill-effects do the feelings of anger, resentment, and hostility have on your heart?

- A study in *Circulation*[17] found that more hostile people were three times more likely to have a heart attack.
- A study in *Archives of Internal Medicine*[18] found that medical students who became angry quickly were three times more likely to develop premature heart disease and had a five times greater chance of having a heart attack.
- Studies show[19] anger and frustration can trigger atrial fibrillation, arrhythmias[20] that can potentially be fatal, leading to sudden cardiac death.

Conversely, people who can constructively cope[21] with their anger have lower resting blood pressures. Our anger, hostilities, and resentments have a direct correlation to our stress levels. Over time, this heightened state of fight-or-flight adds more wear-and-tear on our hearts and health than we want. For example, anger causes hormonal changes,[22] releasing stress hormones—like cortisol and adrenaline—which cause increased heart rate, cholesterol, and blood pressure.

Stress and anger also cause blood vessels to not function properly. A new area of research suggests stress leads to chronic inflammation[23] that results in dysfunction of blood vessels and can cause heart disease.

Plus, these harmful emotions can negatively affect and even compromise our immune system's[24] ability to fight off infections, even cancerous cells. Therefore, if you can find room to forgive others as well as yourself, you will have more reason to smile, feel better and look better for it too!

Stress and Music Do Not Mix

For virtually instant stress relief, turn on some tunes, sing, or hum along, and let the sound of music replace those anxious thoughts. It's amazing how powerful music can be in adjusting our attitudes and gaining a new perspective on what stresses us out. Studies corroborate[25] what most of us feel: Music is a great stress reliever [26] that makes us happy.

While I was on faculty at the University of Maryland School of Medicine, one of my colleagues published a study that found that when you listen to joyful music that you like, your blood vessels dilate, allowing for increased blood flow to the heart and throughout the body. In other words, listening to music can promote heart health.[27]

While listening to music can help you live longer, singing can improve your mood and memory.[28] In a fascinating television segment on CBS's show *60 Minutes*, viewers could literally watch the late legendary crooner Tony Bennett, who was suffering from Alzheimer's, change his demeanor from a blank stare of dementia to happy expression when he heard certain music and started singing. Additionally, even though he often could not recall the day of week or his address, upon hearing instrumental background music from one of his song's, he can start singing without forgetting a single word of the lyrics.

Music has a way of lighting up the brain, and singing along or dancing can be one of the best things you can do for your mental health. Music activates coordination, timing, and memory and fosters friendship, not to mention improving mood and lowering stress.[29] I've experienced this phenomenon at home. My husband works with a Wall Street firm that puts him in meetings and on calls all day long. To take his mind off all of it after work, he goes out on the back deck and turns up his favorite music. Pretty quickly, his stress levels return to baseline as he relaxes to the sound waves.

Listening to music is a simple, cathartic way to regain focus and settle down. It's so simple that we can forget how powerful it is—and you don't even need speakers or equipment. Nearly everyone has access to music now with smart phones. Even just humming[30] can reduce your stress by enhancing the parasympathetic nervous system and slowing down your sympathetic activation of the fight-or-flight response. I know this is true for me; when I hum or sing along with music, it lifts my stress and worries as well as making me feel joyful. It's just like the lyrics from Earth, Wind & Fire's 1975 album *Gratitude*, their hit song "Sing a Song," that tells you to just start singing and it will lift your spirits.

Sleep Away Stress

Increased acute and chronic stress can both lead to problems sleeping,[31] which in turn leads to increased stress. It's a vicious cycle. Adults who sleep less than 7 to 8 hours [32] a night report higher stress levels. Lack of sleep and sleep disorders are common; About 50 to 70 million Americans[33] have chronic, or ongoing, sleep deficiency. This can lead to both physical and mental health conditions, increased risk for injuries, loss of productivity at work and home, increased motor vehicle crashes, as well as a greater likelihood of death. Some studies[34] cite the economic impact to be around $100 billion dollars lost annually due to decrease in productivity, increase in medical expenses, sick leave and property damage from accidents—all related to lack of sleep.

Sleep is a key[35] to ensuring proper cognitive and behavior function, as well as regulation of our metabolism. It serves to restore and repair our brain and body from the day's activities. When we lose sleep, we lose brain power and hence, stress levels increase. But the opposite is also true, when we get enough sleep, we think better, feel better, and react to stress better.

Science shows that sleep gives the brain time to process what we've learned, which translates into increased memory. On the other hand, sleep deprivation affects other body functions; it wears down our immune system[36] and causes a vicious cycle of releasing cortisol, which then turns on our fight-or-flight sympathetic hormonal responses,[37] increasing the risk of high blood pressure and heart disease.

Lack of sleep and its ensuing stress even contributes to obesity[38] from increased levels of hormones like ghrelin, which increases appetite and decreases levels of the hormone leptin, which tells you when you are full and to stop eating, as well causing insulin resistance and increased risk of diabetes.

So how do you break this cycle and get some ZZZs? New evidence shows that slow-wave sleep from napping can keep our brain working and solving problems. Researchers at the University of California-Berkeley[39] found that a one-hour nap can boost and restore brain power and memory. In the study, 39 healthy volunteers in two groups—naps and no-naps—had a grueling set of facts and information taught to them at 2:00 p.m. The nap group napped for 1.5 hours. Then at 6:00 p.m. each group had new learning exercises. They found that the nap group not only did better with learning things at 6:00 p.m., but they also performed better than earlier in the day! Researchers also found that the memory restorative napping doesn't have to be long or deep sleep; it occurred at a specific stage of sleep called Stage 2 non-REM (rapid eye movement, that occurs during dreaming), which is between deep sleep and REM. The bottom line is: Try to get as much sleep as you can, but if need be, just take a nap!

Laugh It Off

Along with being kind to yourself and building your self-esteem, a terrific way to reduce stress, is to not take yourself so seriously. You should be able to give yourself a break and laugh at yourself, faults and all. If you can find the humor in a stressful situation, then you can release the grip of stress. I hope my story has shown that, even though I'm a perfectionist, I just don't take myself too seriously. I'm my own best critic and always think good is not good enough. So, I laugh at myself; otherwise I would be stressed out all the time.

Give yourself permission to laugh it off. After all, the saying, "Laughter is the best medicine," is actually backed by science.[40] And seriously, this is no joke; laughing has healing powers![41] It can diffuse stress and help your mental health but also has physiological benefits. A good belly laugh brings in oxygen to stimulate all the organs, dampens the flight-or-fight response, and dilates blood vessels to lower blood pressure.[42] It has a similar beneficial effect as exercise on the heart.[43]

Laughing can release our internal opioids, endorphins, and increases dopamine, our feel-good neurotransmitters, along with increased serotonin levels, which can battle anxiety and depression to help us feel better.[44] Stimulation of our endocannabinoid system (ECS) also interacts with those areas of the brain[45] and the neurotransmitters related to emotions and happiness; after all, our internal cannabinoid molecule is call anandamide. It was literally named after the Sanskrit word for bliss, *ānanda*; it is our internal bliss molecule. Therefore, it is not surprising that many people who use cannabis, which stimulates our ECS, often have fits of laughter. And laughter has been shown to relieve pain, probably related to stimulation of our endorphins and our ECS.[46]

Long-term laughing and a sense of humor can bolster our immune system[47] by inducing our natural killer (NK) cells, which can destroy infected and disease cells, even cancer cells. One study[48] even showed that laughing can be a food substitute to help you lose weight! We have all heard of emotional eating, and if laughter can lift your mood, maybe you won't reach for those potato chips and ice cream. While I am not saying laughter is the miracle cure, the benefits are undeniable. And as we age, stress comes in new varieties.

What we worried about in our young adulthood can seem funny to us as we age. Those things just don't matter like they once did. That's the perspective we need to realize. What you're going through now could be quite funny later too. So, when you are stressed, find perspective and the humor in your situation. I know it may be easier said than done.

You might try watching a comedy instead of a suspenseful, stress-inducing movie. Seek out jokes and welcome the humor in life.

My son loves to poke fun at my vanity. When we got our dog, I suggested we get her trained for agility contests. But my son thought we should get her trained as a cadaver dog, saying, "Mom, you use so much Botox. In case your face gets too frozen, we may need a way to make sure you're not dead!" This cracked me up!

By not taking ourselves too seriously, I believe we teach ourselves resilience. Plus, it gives us a funny story to tell later. So lighten up!

Cut Out Clutter

Want to relieve stress, save time, and possibly make money in one shot? Here's one of my favorite things to do when I'm feeling stressed. I organize my closet. Or I'll clean off my desk, sort and file paperwork, or get rid of a bunch of stuff that I just don't need.

Studies show that clutter can negatively affect quality of life.[49] Our homes are an extension of us, and how they look and function is key to our well-being. Clutter is often associated with procrastination.[50] Studies show that a cluttered space is a cluttered mind; clutter affects our ability to think clearly and leads to stress and low energy levels.[51]

Clutter at work[52] negatively impacts our job satisfaction and increases job-related relationship tensions and occupational stress. There is continuum, from simple clutter to the pathological psychiatric condition of hoarding. Hoarding is a form of anxiety and obsessive-compulsive disorder.[53] This is an extreme situation where nothing can be discarded, even scraps of paper with no purpose or meaning, and there is severe emotional distress just thinking about discarding these items. This condition often requires psychiatric help and medication to overcome. Additionally, there can be potential physical consequences for hoarders living in dangerous, unsanitary conditions, so it is important to get help.

For simple clutter, though, it just feels great to reorganize a closet or room or clean off your desk. You know where things are, and there's a sense of gratefulness for what you have.

Clutter can either cause stress or reflect having too much stress. Studies[54] find that being surrounded by a cluttered environment can overstimulate the visual cortex, decreasing our ability to concentrate. The more stuff piles up, the more preoccupied our brain becomes; by removing the clutter, our brains can focus again. During stressful times, we often just don't feel like picking things up and putting them away. But when we do, it feels great. The task of cleaning[55] itself can also be a relaxing form of mindfulness. Even something as mundane as washing the dishes can be a stress-relieving practice.[56] I know that for me, I always feel better going to bed after I spend time washing, rinsing, and loading the dishwasher, leaving my kitchen clean. There is nothing worse than waking up the next morning with your kitchen a mess and a sink full of dirty dishes.

Something surreal also happens when you cut out the clutter. You examine what is really important to you and what is just being held onto for, perhaps, no real reason at all. We find this when we're moving, right? That's the best part about moving. We must decide what to box, what to give away, and what to throw out. It's cathartic to let stuff go, not to mention the good feeling you get donating items to those who might need them more. When we get to create a new space with everything put away in a tidy, organized fashion and settle into a clutter-free environment, it feels fabulous.

When I was younger, I didn't appreciate how good making a bed can make you feel. I know we sometimes wake up late and don't have time to make the bed, but studies show that those who make their beds feel calmer and more equipped to handle the day.[57] I must have 14 pillows on my bed: decorative ones, fuzzy ones, contrasting ones—all to make my bed appealing. There are days I don't feel like gathering all the pillows and decorating my bed.

During COVID-19, my bedroom was a disaster. It stressed me out. I was studying for my master's in medical cannabis science, earning a living, and caring for my family. My dad, who was living with me during his series of orthopedic surgeries, needed constant care, so my living room looked more like a hospital room with all kinds of medications, IVs, and other crap all over. I get a nervous tic just thinking about it now. I noticed it was upping the anxiety that I already had worrying about his health. Everything piled higher and higher as the days and weeks passed. But finally, when I'd had enough and cut out the clutter, I felt great. It was a minor accomplishment with huge rewards.

If you're savvy, you can even turn your clutter into cash. These days you can sell your extra stuff online. It's not that hard with Facebook Marketplace, Poshmark, or Rebag. You can actually harness your stress while getting some extra cash at the same time. Cutting the clutter can also save you money, especially if your stuff is sitting storage with a monthly payment. How often do we ever revisit the storage unit we're renting and actually clean them out?

Cutting out the clutter is so important that I recommend taking vacation time off, if you have it, to clear out your house. It can be as relaxing as going on a vacation. And, when you get everything cleared out, your house looks great, you know where everything is, you've given stuff away, maybe made some extra cash, and it really feels wonderful. A happy, clutter-free house is a happy life!

Get High on Nature

I'm one of these people who loves to read and learn about nature. It fascinates me. I even subscribe to *National Geographic*.

When I was a little kid, I loved watching those shows like *Mutual of Omaha's Wild Kingdom*, although it was very distressing to watch the animals kill each other. I always wondered, *Why isn't someone intervening to save them?* That's probably why I have a small home but on 15 acres surrounded by the woods. I used to walk my beloved baby girl, my labradoodle, a couple of times a day as an excuse to get some fresh air, natural sunlight, and a feeling of being immersed in nature.

I highly recommend getting high on nature. There's serenity waiting for us in nature. It's the same powerful/powerless feeling we get when we're near the ocean or looking up at monumental mountains; it puts life into proper perspective. Sometimes I'll just sit on my back deck in the evenings and watch the beautiful little owls sitting in a tree, or the woodpeckers in the woods. I can see the graceful bats coming and going. I also love to watch the foxes, rabbits, and deer in my wooded backyard. It's so beautiful and calming living here, and yet only 30 minutes from the city.

Spending time in nature lowers stress and delivers a wide range of psychological and physiological health benefits. Mounting scientific research[58] suggests that spending two hours in nature a week promotes good health and psychological well-being. According to this study, it doesn't matter if it is a long visit or several shorter visits every week. It can lower blood pressure and stress hormone levels, reduce nervous system arousal, enhance immune system function, increase self-esteem, reduce anxiety, and improve mood.

This study corroborates previous research that finds people living in and around greener urban areas have less cardiovascular disease,[59] obesity,[60] diabetes,[61] and mental distress,[62] and even lower mortality rates.[63] Although the researchers acknowledge that time spent in nature is often associated with higher levels of physical activity, the research indicated some benefits cannot be due solely to activity. It doesn't even matter whether you are walking through a wooded trail or just sitting in a park and taking it in, being outside in nature is beneficial to your mental and physical health.

Researchers out of Sweden[64] conducted an interesting study comparing stress levels associated with an urban environment, forest, and park settings. They sought to identify if adding urban green spaces to city planning would help reduce stress. They looked at experiencing "nature and green spaces" using virtual reality, accompanied with olfactory (smells) and auditory stimuli. No surprise, they found a link between physical stress reduction and the perceived nature spaces. Surprisingly, however, they found stress levels did not correlate with how spectacular the imagery looked; it appeared that olfactory stimuli were more effective at reducing stress than visual stimuli. But even urban green spaces can elicit stress-reducing effects, according to the study. So city-dwellers don't have an excuse not to get to some green spaces and parks within their cities.

It's not surprising that the Japanese would value time in nature and the forest. Most of the island, 75 percent, is made up of uninhabitable mountains and forest, but the majority of Japan's population is crowded into densely populated urban areas like Tokyo, which is listed as one of the world's most crowded cities.

A study[65] done in Japan found that being in nature and forest settings promotes lower stress hormone levels and lower sympathetic nerve activity; time in nature was also associated with lower blood pressure and heart rate when compared to city environments. There is even a name for this time in nature in Japanese: *shinrin-yoku*, forest bathing. The positive effects can come from merely sitting passively in natural settings. So when you're feeling particularly stressed out, go experience nature—and enjoy the sights, sounds and smells.

Soak the Stress Away

Speaking of forest bathing, one of the best investments I ever made when doing my master bedroom/bathroom renovation was buying a great soaking tub. The return on that investment has been hours of soothing away my stress in a hot tub. I love it. I know some people don't like tubs because they feel like they are bathing in their own filth, but I say, "Shower off first then, you can use the bathtub for relaxation," if that worries you!

Some people use bath salts and/or bubbles with scents like lavender, whose scent comes from a terpene called linalool, also found in cannabis, and has a calming effect. But even without those, I love getting into a tub, soaking, and closing my eyes. I like to go underwater and listen to the rhythm of my heartbeat. I feel like I'm soaking away my stress, as well as tuning everything else out and using the time for just me to relax.

Studies show that taking a soaking immersion bath,[66] or even a shower,[67] is beneficial to your mental and physical health. Baths can help with anxiety and depression by releasing endorphins. They can reduce our stress hormone, cortisol. Studies[68] find that a warm shower or soak before bed can improve the quality of sleep and help with insomnia.

And just like stress reduction seen in green spaces (nature), there is also associated stress reductions with outdoor blue spaces,[69] such as lakes, oceans, and rivers. So just spending time near water outdoors and/or soaking in it indoors helps relieve stress and puts us in a much better mood.

Lean on Me

It's important find your support systems so that you realize you are not alone. So often, we can get caught up in the stressors of life that we withdraw or escape with a bottle of wine. This is definitely not a healthy way to manage or harness stress.

While loneliness is not technically a medical condition, it has become a widespread problem in the US that has been taken up by our Surgeon

General.[70] People who reported high levels of loneliness[71] and social isolation have an increased risk of both mental and physical health problems. A Harvard University report[72] found that 61percent of young adults ages 18 to 25 as well as 39 percent of the general population reported serious feelings of loneliness, which was worsened since the pandemic.

According to the CDC,[73] not only are people at increased risk for mental health conditions such as addiction, depression, anxiety, and suicide, they are also at increased risk for other medical problems such as heart disease, stroke, diabetes, and early death. A recent study[74] found that having a support system to talk things over during a stressful situation can build resilience.

Often the best thing you can do is pick up the phone and reach out to someone who cares. Friends, family, or a therapist can make for an incredible safety net and support system when tough times threaten your internal peace. For me, I would talk things out with my mom. She was a great listener and always brought me back from the moon, helping me get my feet on the ground—emotionally. Since she died, I've learned there are others in my life, to lean on, like my husband or my best friend, who is really more of the sister that I always wanted. I call her daily and this helps me immensely. Describing our feelings about stress makes it more tangible and gives our confidante a chance to participate in possible solutions, or maybe just lend a sympathetic and empathetic ear.

If you feel like you don't have that trusted friend or advisor, you can develop connections with those in other communities. You might try your religious institution, or getting involved with a charity or other special interest support group where you have a common stressor or goal, such as grief management groups or substance abuse programs. Even adopting a pet, which we will discuss coming up, helps with the feelings of isolation. Having these kinds of outlets allows you to let off some steam in a healthy way.

Sweat It Out

The opposite of a calming bubble bath is a sweaty workout that stresses our body, but in a good way. Numerous of studies have shown the many benefits exercises has on the health of the body and mind. We know the obvious benefits exercise has for our physical health, such as cardiovascular health and more, but it is equally important for our mental health.[75] Exercise can reduce stress, anxiety, and depression,[76] and lessen symptoms of low self-esteem and social withdrawal.

Even though I don't really like to exercise, I find it is one of the best stress-relievers—it floods my body with helpful endorphins and endocannabinoids that help me focus and feel better.

We all know we need exercise, so why don't we all do it? We have excuses, but the most common one that I hear from patients (and sometimes from myself) is a lack of time. We simply haven't made it a priority.

If a doctor told you to avoid eating peanuts due to an allergy that could kill you, I'm pretty sure you'd never eat peanuts again. It should be the same with exercise. So I'm prescribing exercise to you right now. But what kind? How much? It depends on your condition, but just start slowly somewhere and somehow that doesn't cause injury.

Moderate physical activity is about 30 minutes per day at least five times a week, and about an hour a day for kids. But studies have shown that doing short bursts of activity throughout your day is cumulative.[77] You can incorporate five to ten minutes of increased activity five times a day, and that can be your 30 minutes. It's been called the "active lifestyle approach."[78] So don't take the elevator at work; take the stairs. Don't circle endlessly for a parking space at the mall; park at the farthest space and walk briskly in and around the mall. You may even find you have more time in the day as you hurry through your errands. Rake the leaves and vacuum like your life depends on it, since it might!

Besides, there's more to exercise than improving your heart and relieving stress. I admit I begrudgingly drag myself to the Peleton due to my vanity. The sheer terror of being seen naked does wonders for my commitment to exercise. Whether you do it for your butt or mood, exercise does makes you feel better afterwards. I can't tell whether I'm relieved my exercise session is over or whether my endocannabinoids are really pumping, or both. But truthfully, it doesn't matter. I just know I do feel better.

Exercise can also make you smarter. Scientists have found that physical activity exerts an effect on the brain through neurogenesis, the creation of new neurons.[79] The new neurons are created in the hippocampus, the center of learning and memory in the brain. This restorative effect is particularly relevant to women because the brain starts to lose nerve tissue beginning at age 30. Aerobic exercise, for example, reinforces neural connections by increasing the number of dendrite connections between neurons, creating a denser network, which is then better able to process and store information. It is believed to help lower the risk of dementia and cognitive decline as we age.[80] Studies show[81] that it can help reduce further cognitive decline and behavioral problems in people who already have impairment or dementia.

Physical activity can also decrease your risk of cancer on the molecular level. A Danish study[82] showed it decreased the incidents of cancer and prevented progression via tumor intrinsic factors that inhibit tumor growth. Another study[83] found a correlation between increased physical activity and exercise with reduced risk of developing certain cancers, such as colorectal and breast cancer. Continuing to exercise with a cancer diagnosis has been shown to possibly help with long-term survival, as well as help cancer survivors cope and recover better during their treatment.

Obviously, exercise helps maintain a healthy weight, too, which is critical for our physical and mental health, as well as our self-esteem. Excess weight in the mid-section is especially dangerous; it can lead to increased risk of death regardless of total body fat.[84] Abdominal fat is very metabolically active, influencing hormones like cortisol, insulin, and estrogen, which can increase risk of cardiovascular disease and diabetes as well as stimulate cancer cell growth in cancers like breast and colon. Even losing as little as 5 to 10 percent of your body weight can decrease belly fat and increase your odds of living longer and healthier.[85]

Keeping active is critical for a healthy lifestyle, especially as we age. It is important to do a combination of different exercises. Cardio includes brisk walks, running, swimming, and biking and is good for heart, circulation, and lungs. Mix that up with a couple days of strength training, starting with your own body weight; moving on to weights helps develop and maintain muscle mass, strength, and bone density, which all decrease as we age. This will help with balance and coordination to prevent falls. Flexibility training increases the overall range of motion of a joint and its surrounding muscles during a passive movement or stretching to reduce the risk of injury. Flexibility is also critical for balance and muscle tone as we age.

Contrary to the title of this book, exercise may be one occasion when you can let others see you sweat! That's good for you because it's a good indicator that your heart rate has been elevated, and you're burning calories!

Have Sex Instead!

There's nothing like a good orgasm. Sex is a natural way to reduce stress and improve sleep. It has many other wonderful health benefits as well, so it's important to cultivate a healthy sex life. I know for me, it's easier to eat less at dinner and give up dessert when I know I'll be naked later. So it can reduce caloric intake as well!

Physiologically, sex can reduce stress and boost your mood by stimulating parts of the brain that increase the release of neurotransmitters like dopamine,[86] the feel-good chemical from the brain's reward center. Sexual arousal can also increase our endorphin levels,[87] which is great for blocking pain. Sex also increases levels of our internal cannabinoids, such as anandamide (our bliss molecule) and 2AG.[88] Physical touch during sex causes the release of oxytocin,[89] often called the love and cuddle hormone. This hormone increases social connection and bonding and is also released in women during breast-feeding. The hormone prolactin is also released,[90] which is responsible for that relaxed, satisfied feeling and sleepiness afterward. Touching, hugging, and sexual intimacy can also reduce our stress hormones, such as adrenaline and cortisol.[91]

Sex can also improve our skin! It boosts sex hormones like estrogen, which can improve skin quality,[92] and increases blood flow to skin, giving it that gorgeous glow. Sex also helps prevent pimples and other skin conditions such as dermatitis and psoriasis, because it reduces stress hormone—such as cortisol—levels that contribute to it.

People who have sex at least three times a week can look up to ten years younger than those who make love less frequently, according to researchers at the Royal Edinburgh Hospital.[93] This lovely side effect is partly because sex helps trigger the production of a human growth hormone that declines as we age, and this hormone can restore tissue, helping us maintain a youthful look.

Sex may not burn a lot of calories, about 150 to 200 an hour,[94] if you can keep it up that long, but it is a nice workout. It's comparable to a brisk walk, but infinitely more fun! Sex raises the heart rate and pumps oxygen around the body and benefits blood pressure, muscle tone, and the cardiovascular system. A study found that men who had sex twice a week had lower risk of developing heart disease.[95]

Sex also benefits the brain's function and health. One study[96] looking at sex in adults between 50 and 89 years old found it improved memory and cognitive function. And another study[97] showed having closeness and more frequent sexual activity with a partner was associated with better performance on memory tests. But taking matters into your own hands does wonders, too.

You don't need a partner to enjoy all of these health benefits, and it can even be more convenient; you don't need to worry about shaving those legs and pits! Masturbation helps you explore your body better to understand what you need from intimacy and how to achieve an orgasm without the worries of how you look or sexually transmitted infections (STI)!

I would be remiss as a woman and physician not to mention that sometimes post-menopausal sex can be painful due to vaginal atrophy and dryness. It is a conversation I have often with women patients when talking about sex, but rubbing a small amount of a topical low-dose estrogen cream around the inner labial folds and just at the opening of the vagina, the most painful area with stretching from sex, can do wonders. There is no risk of breast cancer risk or cardiovascular disease with this form of hormone replacement because the estrogen stays in the vaginal tissue.[98]

Whether you have sex with a partner or by yourself, you can reap the physical benefits along with the emotional well-being associated with it.

Create in the Kitchen

Besides cooking in the bedroom, you can also start cooking in the kitchen to relax and relieve stress. I love to entertain and create healthy dishes. That is an immediate physical health benefit because I like to transform unhealthy fatty and sugary recipes into healthy versions that I don't feel guilty eating. I also love to bake and decorate my breads and desserts. I'll cut out stencils and use powdered sugar or frosting to create amazing-looking items. It gives me a creative outlet when I've got a lot on my mind.

While it can be challenging, I find it very rewarding. It puts you in the present, which is a form of mindfulness that allows you to focus on something other than your worries. A review study[99] looking at cooking in home economic courses corroborates it as a form of mindfulness. And many other studies have shown the importance of mindfulness in stress reduction to both improve mental health and its associated physical health benefits too.[100, 101, 102, 103]

Even if you're already "chief cook and bottle washer" at home and you feel like the kitchen is the last place you want to spend time "relaxing," maybe don't jump out of that proverbial frying pan so quickly. Bad clichés aside, there's plenty of stress-relief when making something delicious and beautiful. Another study revealed that a little creativity in the kitchen can make people happier. That study was published in the *Journal of Positive Psychology*, suggesting that people who frequently take on small, creative projects like baking or cooking report feeling more relaxed and happier in their everyday lives.[104]

It is very satisfying to have a vision, plan out the ingredients, and then execute the plan, overcoming any challenges along the way. I believe cooking can increase confidence, boost self-esteem, and make you feel better. And research backs me up. It has been found to improves self-esteem and quality of life[105] while increasing emotional stability.[106]

Who cares if you try something and it doesn't come out perfectly the first time; you have the chance to do it again. Cooking and baking give you the experience of overcoming failures, an important skill to learn when building resilience. The act of cooking and baking for someone else is also a form of generosity that is very fulfilling. Additionally, cooking with others in the family makes for a great bonding experience, as we share in the rewards from our efforts. I love it when my son comes home from graduate school on the holidays and joins me in the kitchen. We've created some amazing meals, cakes, and pies together. But really the best part is making those memories together.

Creating in the kitchen is one of my favorite ways to harness my stress and turn it into something wonderful and delicious!

Play Around

Kids do not have the market cornered on playing. Adults need to play too. Whether we're playing sports, video games, or board games, or doing puzzles, drawing, painting, or even flower-arranging, we're taking our minds and bodies off stress.

A systematic review study[107] looked at the health benefits of playing board games. Aside from the obvious camaraderie and community-building skills, playing board games was also found to improve cognitive function and decrease symptoms of anxiety, attention deficit hyperactivity disorder (ADHD), and even Alzheimer's disease. Doing puzzles with family members can have similar effects.

Another study published in *Trends in Psychology*[108] looked at college students during the pandemic, a particularly stressful time for students due to social isolation. The researchers found that playing casual video games was an effective stress-reduction strategy similar to mindfulness and medications. In fact, the researchers recommended that these post-secondary institutions consider setting up video game stations in students' common areas. My own son started graduate school in a new town during the pandemic and spent all his time locked in his apartment taking classes and teaching online but was able to blow off steam and de-stress by playing video games.

Getting creative with art is another effective stress reducer. In fact, art therapy is a recognized medical discipline, like occupational therapy. It is used with various psychiatric conditions, such as depression, borderline personality disorder, schizophrenia, and post-traumatic stress-disorder (PTSD),[109] but everyone can benefit from a little artistic play. A study published in the *Journal of American Art Therapy Association* measured cortisol levels in healthy volunteers before and after making art and found statistically significant lower levels of these stress hormones.[110]

If you don't know where to begin with drawing, painting, or sculpting, look no further than the commercial products on the market now. They make both coloring books and Legos for adults, so give one (or both!) a try. You may be surprised by how much fun you have—and how creative you can get!

Get a Dog

My baby girl was a gorgeous black labradoodle with the most soulful eyes and so smart. I loved her. I say it all the time, but I could not have loved her more if I had given birth to her myself. She was the perfect daughter I always wanted but never had. I am not sure I will every fully recover from her death at 14.5 years old due to cancer, malignant melanoma.

Even though I had a childhood dog I loved, it doesn't feel the same. I went off to college and med school when our family dog died. Having a dog as an adult felt different; it really felt like she was my baby—and she was. She made me a better person and it was my honor to care for her. I know some of you can relate to what I'm saying.

I was a neurotic dog mother (no surprise, right?!) and I was proud of it; however, I am still reeling that, as a doctor, I could not save her. I know she was over 14 years old, which is considered old for a big dog, but it felt too soon. She still looked as cute as a damn puppy.

How could I love my dog this much? She loved me unconditionally. When I looked into her eyes, all the problems from the day seemed to fade away. And science backs me up on this, a study[111] found that when dog parents stare into the eyes of their dogs and the dogs stare into their eyes, both release the cuddle-love hormone oxytocin—a similar feedback loop to what is seen between mothers and their infants. So, for those skeptical non-dog people who say our pets only love us because we house and feed them, it's not true. They really do just love us for who we are, family, and their hormones say so! Dogs experience a 130 percent rise in oxytocin while their humans experience a 300 percent rise.

I saw firsthand how my baby girl affected my physical health. I could consistently see a drop in my measured blood pressure when she was sitting next to me and touching me. According to the American Heart Association's statement paper [112] published in their journal, *Circulation,* pets can lower our heart rate, blood pressure, cholesterol, triglycerides, and even blood sugar. Pets can help combat social isolation,[113] with over 36 percent less loneliness reported.

A 2012 review study found that interacting with animals[114] not only reduces anxiety and depression, but it even encourages more positive interactions with other humans too—probably other dog parents at the park! It's amazing how easy it is to strike up a conversation with another dog person. And many men will attest to the fact that a cute dog can be a "chick magnet."

Owning a pet can also prolong your life,[115] with a 24 percent decreased risk in all-cause mortality. Dog parents are more likely to get exercise, spending on average 200 more minutes a week walking than people that don't have a dog, enabling them to meet recommended physical fitness guidelines.[116] However, as we age, we must be careful walking our fur babies. I have seen my fair share of broken hips in the ER from those sudden jerks and turns when squirrel or other dog passes by. But it is no doubt that our pets enrich our lives with their unconditional love that knows no bounds.

Key Takeaways

- Find a female doctor; it will improve your health.
- Learn to use your smile; it a secret weapon.
- Learn to cheer yourself on. You deserve it.

- Learn to forgive others and yourself; its good for your heart.
- Listen to more music; it soothes your stress and makes you happy.
- Get a good night's sleep and consider taking a nap when needed.
- Learn to laugh at yourself, and do not take life too seriously.
- Clean up and organize your house; it will make your feel better.
- Get outdoors more. Enjoying nature will ease your mind and body.
- Take a bath and soak your stresses away.
- Break a sweat exercising; it can help with your mental health too.
- Have more sex either alone or with someone; it will improve your mood.
- Bake something delicious and beautiful and then share it with someone.
- Color or build a Lego project. Adults can reap the benefits of play too!
- Get a dog (or cat or any pet); it will enhance your life immeasurably!

Chapter 7

Ways to Steward Stress

While I've learned many things to do to harness stress, I've also learned many things *not* to do to better manage my stress. This is not a list of ways to get your partner or spouse to do things for you, although that would be nice. My goal is to encourage women to give themselves a friggin' break. The fantasy we see on TV of busy career women seamlessly balancing their careers and home lives is not realistic. We all have stresses and struggles to deal with; however, putting our worries into perspective really helps, especially when we look at what is happening in our world today.

I often need to check myself and consciously take stock of my concerns in the greater scheme of life. I realize that we can be influenced by circumstances and people we cannot always control. Despite the tragedies we hear about in the news daily, which can make our woes seem inconsequential, we still have our own stressful demands on our time and attention. We need to make a living, run errands for the family, be on-call for family emergencies, keep the house clean, make dinner, and do the laundry. And when we read magazines or see TV shows showing the ease with which these supposed women goddesses do it all, we feel less than. It's enough to cry yourself to sleep some nights.

I know life throws us all fastballs at times, but at least we're in the game. We can still control the words that we say to ourselves and to others. That matters, because how we think and talk to ourselves affects how we feel and our behaviors. This means we can control our thoughts, beliefs, and behaviors. And we must tell ourselves, that we cannot control people or certain life situations, so we have to learn to let those things go.

This chapter is about letting go of the things we cannot control and instead, using each situation as motivation to carry us forward. We are women. We are capable of great things, and we can't let the stressful situations in our lives hold us back.

So cut yourself some slack. Try not to overschedule yourself; set your limits and learn to say no so you can make time for yourself.

DON'T SWEAT THE SMALL STUFF

I can't say it enough, when stressed about something, I would always hear my mom's voice asking, "Is this really worth getting cancer or a heart attack over?" She was not a physician, but she was right. She knew there was a link to stress and health! We've already discussed how chronic stress can affect heart disease.[1] A study found that the area in the brain that processes fear and anxiety, called the amygdala, can trigger a cascade of events causing artery inflammation leading to blockage and a heart attack once activated.[2,3] Chronic stress can also affect cancer outcomes through cortisol levels. And certain white blood cells found that can increase the incidence of spread through metastasis and poorer survival rates.[4]

As an ER doc and a certified germaphobe who stresses about every little bacterium, virus, or other pathogen that could possibly invade my life, you can imagine the stress I had during a shift covered in blood, pus, and other bodily fluids. During my residency, I separated my normal clothes from my scrubs and washed my scrubs at a laundromat—not my building's laundry room. My scrubs never really made it through the door; I often came home in the middle of the night after an exhausting shift and would take off my shoes and scrubs in the hallway since no one else was up and about then, and put them in separate bags before walking into my apartment barefoot in my underwear.

Once, at 3:00 a.m. after a late shift, the door shut and locked with my keys in my bag just inside the door! There I was in the middle of the hallway in my underwear. Humiliated, I walked myself to the superintendent's apartment; he took one look at me and said he didn't even want to know the situation before sleepily walking me back to open my apartment door. All my friends, family, colleagues, and I had a good laugh about it! The situations being a germaphobe can get you into! I used to shriek when my husband put his suitcase on the bed, or when he would sit on our bed, even on top of the comforter, in his blue jeans or outside clothes. I really should have grown up in Japan, making sure everyone takes off their outside shoes before entering my house.

In an ironic twist, though, after joining our family, our beautiful baby labradoodle got full access to my bed and all furniture regardless of whether she had been chasing deer or rolling around in the dirt and leaves. I'd let her come home and roll all over my sheets, no less, below the comforters! My boundless love for her did not set off my germaphobe-meter, which makes me wonder, *Am I guilty of sweating the small stuff?* She was allowed to bring in any pathogens into our home and it was okay by me! So, where's the line?

I have to say, after we got her, I did cut my hubby a little more slack about sitting on the bed. There are stresses that we must let go of sometimes. And certainly, in situations we cannot do anything about, why waste our time, energy, or even our health on getting worked up? We all need to find our own line in the sand; otherwise we will get too stressed from sweating the small stuff.

The next time you feel stress coming on, try asking yourself, "Is this really worth jeopardizing my health and sanity to get stressed out about? Is getting all worked up really doing anybody, including me, any good? If I let this go, will the consequences really hurt me or my ability to live my life?"

In other words, become a student of yourself. Monitor your thoughts before making rash decisions. Learn your triggers and learn to see them coming. Soon, you'll be able to see that many irritations in life are only temporary. There's no purpose in stressing about things outside of our control, and that goes for boneheads cutting you off on the highway. You can either give them the finger and try to race pass them with some road rage, which in today's world may have serious, even deadly, consequences, or just keep your eyes on the road ahead and settle into the driver's seat with the radio turned up.

DON'T MAKE RETAIL THERAPY YOUR GO-TO

I get it, I really do. There are times that I feel my stress level and anxiety decreasing as I peruse the aisles of inside my favorite department store. I even love walking in a beautiful, upscale grocery store, thinking about the meals I can prepare or if I want to bring home a delicious, ready-made one. There is a wonderful deli and store in New York called Zabar's that I love to go to. It's relaxing for me to go one of my favorite stores and pick up something to eat or wear. That's when we can feel in control, at peace, and have power. Heck, I'm guilty of buying a few extra sets of a clothing item that I love just in case I lose one or it wears out.

I remember in college, on a tight budget, if I had a choice between buying dinner or buying an item of clothing, I'd choose the new clothing item every time. I guess you could call that a "true retail diet" because it was an effective way for me to lose weight and look good in those new duds!

But seriously there is a danger in retail therapy. Buying more stuff isn't always the best answer to relieving stress. In fact, it can become a bad habit, leading to maxed-out credit cards, which can then cause more stress and health issues as we age.[5] According to the American Public Health Association,[6] household debt can cause anxiety and depression. It is even harmful to your physical well-being by contributing to high blood pressure and heart disease. If you're spending too much money, especially on credit, it can cause a strain on your relationship. Financial problems can negatively affect the quality of your relationship with your partner.[7] According to the American Psychological Association,[8] over one-third of couples reported money issues as a problem in their relationship. Other studies find these arguments tend to be the most intense and often unresolved problems that couples can have.[9] So if you believe this applies to your relationship, it may be something you need professional help with before there is irreparable damage.

One of the worst feelings is buyer's remorse. When you feel lousy about spending too much on something or just buying something you don't need, you often wind up not liking it. Wasting money can be very stressful. Those irresistible Black Friday deals might come with a bigger price tag than you think! The economic climate, unemployment rates, rising energy and food prices, along with rising credit card debt can all take a toll on your health.[10]

Ailments such as ulcers, migraines, anxiety and panic attacks, backaches, severe depression, and heart attacks are linked to increased stress related to increased debt.[11] This corroborates other studies that show this type of high interest debt is bad for mental health.[12] It found that as interest rates increased, so did the borrower's stress, and that changing interest rates pose a threat to the mental health of those heavily indebted. This can lead to anger and other negative emotions that can trigger anxiety and hostility from economic worries that in turn can cause arrhythmias and irregular heartbeats.[13]

Therefore, if your stress is related to debt, be strong before you hit the computer for those pre-Black Friday or Cyber-Monday deals or set your alarm for 3:00 a.m. to be there when the doors open. The ephemeral rush you get when shopping quickly fades when you get the credit card bill. Think hard about whether you're putting yourself deeper in debt. You must exert your power and control.

Try shopping without buying anything. You'd be surprised at how good it can feel to just browse without spending or wasting money on something you probably don't need. Or try shopping your closet; I bet there's something in the back you've forgotten about that you might have loved when you bought it and it can feel new again! Hell, I hate to admit it, but I have found things tucked in the back of my closet with the price tag still on them, never even worn, yet still in style!

DON'T SELF-MEDICATE

Here's some advice that could save your life: If you're turning to drugs, alcohol, and even food to self-medicate your stress and anxiety, you're heading into dangerous territory. The fact is that always using a substance as a crutch can make you vulnerable to addiction, which only makes matters worse.[14]

It's one thing to have a glass of wine with dinner on occasion, but if you find that every single day or night you "need" that extra glass to relax, then you're setting yourself up for an unhealthy habit that can cause a lot more harm than good. This kind of habit can escalate and lead to a physical dependence and emotional crutch that make matters worse, increasing your stress and anxiety and in a viscous cycle leading to depression.[15,16]

By writing this book, I hope to equip you with ways to deal with your stresses, even harness them. But escaping, withdrawing, or avoiding stress only manifests more stress! We have to find healthy ways to cope, then have the self-esteem, resilience, and resourcefulness to face the stress—instead of losing it temporarily at the bottom of a bottle.

You probably don't need a doctor to tell you that abusing alcohol and drugs is bad for your mental, physical, and relational health. I've seen it destroy lives of patients and their families and, unfortunately, I have seen enough overdoses to last me a lifetime. It's never pretty and never the answer to the problem.

Other types of compulsive behaviors can also become destructive to your health and relationships. I'm referring to behavioral addictions like gambling, pornography, and even "emotional eating."

While I was working on my master's degree, I was juggling my work, family, and home life and was not always harnessing my stress in the best ways. So I found myself eating a lot more than normal, as I felt stressed. Every time I stepped on the scale, I could literally see the stress adding up.

There is a link between stress and overeating.[17] Overeating is a known risk factor for obesity and binge eating disorder (BED.)[18] The stress fight-or-flight response was an evolutionary advantage at one point, and eating was a part of that. First, we need the energy to fight or run, and as hunters and gatherers, we ate when there was food—the next meal was never guaranteed.

Our species back then, as well as all others, were more at risk for starvation than being overweight, so it was an adaptation to eat around times of stress,[19] but not actually when we were running from that mastodon! Our cravings during stress are usually for consuming comfort foods that are high in calories, fats, and sugars we crave, probably because of their high energy source. In fact, it's called hedonic feeding under stress, and studies with animals have found a feedback loop in the brain.[20] Not only does it evolutionarily provide energy during our flight-or-fight response, but food also triggers other areas in the brain, such as the reward center, to release the feel-good neurotransmitter dopamine to mitigate negative feelings.[21]

I recognized my stress as a signal to eat more and decided to make some changes. Watch for these signals, and have the courage to be honest with yourself to take action. But as I always say, don't beat yourself up about it. Overindulging, especially with food, is hard-wired in us; it's not lack of will power. Today, we physicians realize that obesity is a disease, and there is medical help with new medications that people can get to combat it.

DON'T DIET

Ditch the diet. It seems like every January that a new diet shows up promising to be the quick-fix to lose weight and look great. I know because I've tried virtually all of them. If I'm addicted to anything, it might be to dieting.

Honestly, I try every diet that comes along; I tell myself it's for research. But frankly it's amusing; it keeps things interesting. I've run the gamut from the grapefruit-and-cabbage diet to my own homemade watermelon-only diet (that caused me to pass out as camp counselor), through my no-carb phase— or as my five-year-old described it to me at the time, "an Adkins nutcase."

My nana was one of the first crusaders of Weight Watchers, back in the 60s when it started, with founder Jean Nidetch's biggest disciple and largest franchisee in Michigan's Florine Marks! Before anyone really talked about glycemic indexes, as a six-year-old I could tell you how bananas had more sugar than apples. And I can still hear Nana's voice again saying, "Chickadee (that's what she called me), you're not fat, but you don't want to get that way, either, so learn to watch yourself."

Sadly, with social media today, it's worse; studies have found that the average six-year-old girl thinks about her weight and may have even tried dieting.[22] Despite my mother's well-meaning mantra of self-acceptance that she had tried to instill in me, probably from fighting all those battles herself with my nana, her mother, my teenage years were riddled with self-doubt and fears of being fat. Looking back, there was nothing further from the truth, yet I disguised my physique with the baggiest clothes! So, this learning to "watch myself" for some 40 or 50 years, which actually caused an unhealthy obsessive relationship with my weight, food, and dieting. A wrong number on that scale in the morning could crush my spirit for the whole day or even week. And I am still a work in progress with self-acceptance with respect to my weight.

It took years into adulthood to learn and firmly believe that we need to ditch these extreme diets and instead maintain a healthy lifestyle. Studies show that severe restriction seen in dieting can lead to eating disorders in about a quarter of dieters.[23] Diets do more harm than good.[24] Time and time again, I've seen how dieting can result in short-term weight loss but fail to have long-term effects.

Diets are stressful because they are often too restrictive and force the body to change the way it uses nutrition and calories. There's no way we're going to keep up and we fall off the diet wagon and start the cyclical yo-yo dieting, with up-and-down weight loss that can be even more harmful to your health.[25] Losing and gaining weight repeatedly has been found to increase inflammation, which puts us at risk for diabetes and heart disease.

In fact, a *New England Journal of Medicine*[26] study, people who yo-yo dieted had a 78 percent higher risk of developing new onset diabetes, a 117 percent higher risk of having a heart attack, a 136 percent higher risk of having a stroke and a 124 percent higher risk of dying.

Finding a varied nutrient-dense diet is critical to a healthy lifestyle. Drastic, highly restrictive diets—that cut out or malign one food category—and unrealistic time frames to meet weight goals are not maintainable or healthy. Set realistic goals that can be done in a realistic time frame. I want to give you few guidelines that I have learned to live by. I hate the cliché, but it is true that moderation is the key.

- You may need to learn to cook a little so that you know what is in your food; you can use healthy ingredients, such as healthy fats with a tasty variety of spices and ingredients you can pronounce, because processed prepared foods that have a lot of ingredients and sound like a chemical PhD thesis have big health risks.[27]
- Learn to enjoy a wide variety of brightly colored fresh fruits and vegetables; it's called eating the rainbow. Colorful fruits and vegetables have the healthiest phytonutrients.[28] Shop more around the edges of the grocery store where the fresh foods are usually found, instead of the middle aisles, which have more processed foods.
- Don't be hard on yourself for "blowing it" once in a while. It can be a nice reward to enjoy a cookie or chocolate; however, this does not include emptying a tub of ice cream or a whole sleeve of Oreos. I like the 80 to 85 percent versus 20 to 15 percent rule: The majority of the time you eat healthy, but occasionally let yourself splurge, especially when you are out at a fabulous restaurant.
- Read labels for calorie counts, serving sizes, sugar and fat content, as well as other unhealthy ingredients. This will familiarize you with healthy portions as well as daily calorie limits. Spending a week or two writing down what you eat, you might surprise yourself with how often and how much you eat. This awareness makes it easier to stay within some limits.

- Avoid mindless eating. Studies show that when deliberately sitting and enjoying our food, we consume fewer calories and feel fuller after.[29] Mindless eating includes eating and/or snacking while on the go or while watching television or a movie. This often includes unhealthy choices such as chips, crackers, cookies, and processed foods. Writing down everything you eat for a couple of weeks will clue you into how many times a day you mindlessly grab a few chips or cookies, because it adds up.
- Enjoy the fine art, and challenge, of substituting healthy choices for bad ones, such as colorful, high-fiber mixed berries and a little whipped cream for dessert instead of cake or cookies, or 70 percent dark chocolate instead of milk chocolate, which has more sugar, less fiber, and less of the healthy antioxidant cacao,[30] which has been shown in moderation to have health benefits.
- Making substitutions in recipes for healthy options is important, too, such as cutting the sugar and adding fruit instead. But beware of artificial sweeteners, also called non-nutritive sweeteners; they are in practically everything today and studies[31] have shown they increase insulin resistance, the very thing it was intended to bypass in diabetics. Frequent use from an early age causes an insensitivity to sweetness,[32] causing you to eat and crave more food and sweets. Our bodies can't adjust to taking in something that tastes sweet but has no calories or nutrition. Additionally, artificial sweeteners[33] negatively affect our gut bacteria and microbiome, which can contribute to obesity. They have also been shown to increase our cardiovascular risk and death.
- Get to know your "carbs." Not all carbohydrates[34] were made equal, which means you have to choose wisely between the good, the bad, and the truly ugly. You might know that carbs come in two forms: simple and complex. What does that really mean? Simple carbs are chemically made of one or two sugars (which includes most all processed and "white" foods: table sugar, syrup, honey, and so on), and are broken down and absorbed quickly into the bloodstream. They are often classified by their glycemic index,[35] which is dependent on how refined or processed the carbohydrates are and a measure of how fast they release glucose when metabolized. Simple carbs have a high glycemic index because they produce a rapid increase in blood sugar; it happens very quickly, and you can get a sugar high and then a crash. Complex carbs like those found in some fruits and vegetables are mixed with fiber and contain longer chains of sugar molecules; they are digested more slowly and have a steadier release of glucose into the blood stream. Understanding this is important in helping regulate your blood sugar. Only so much sugar is needed to replace the sugar (glycogen) stored in your muscle and liver. When eaten in excess, sugar goes into our fat cells. A fat cell can swell to *50 times its original size* to accommodate

more fat.[36] Stay away from refined carbs with less fiber to feel and look better over the long haul.

- The types of fats in your diet are important too. Healthy unsaturated fats are the best.[37] In the 1960s, it was actually the sugar industry that vilified all fats,[38] related fat intake to heart disease, and the "low fat" craze began, which replaced fats with sugars, and over the next several decades it actually increased our obesity epidemic and its associated metabolic problems, like diabetes and heart disease, the very medical problems that it was intended to help.

- Without a doubt, unsaturated fats are part of a heart-healthy diet.[39] They are found in some fruits and vegetables like nuts, olives, avocados, and lean proteins such as fish. And this is why time and time again when science assesses the types of diets that are the healthiest and should be a lifestyle choice. They are a heavily plant-based diet[40] and/or one like the Mediterranean diet[41,42] found in many blue zones,[43] regions around the world where people live longer and healthier lives than average.

Maintain a healthy lifestyle with activity and a diet focused heavily on a plant-based foods, a lot of colorful fruits, vegetables, nuts, and whole grains along with lean proteins such as fish, but also consider trying to limit ultra-processed foods, unhealthy fats, and sugars. This will not only help you maintain a healthy weight, but it will improve important markers such as cholesterol and triglyceride levels, that will in turn lower the risks of developing high blood pressure, diabetes, and cardiovascular disease.

DON'T WORK YOURSELF TO DEATH

The United States leads the way as a no-vacation nation. America is one of the few westernized countries without government-sanctioned, paid vacation days.[44] Only three-quarters of US employers offer paid holiday leave, and when they do, it is usually only 10 days.[45] Most European governments sanction a full month: Spain and Germany offer 34 days of holiday; France and Italy have 30 days; the United Kingdom gives 28 days; and Scandinavian countries pay for 25 days. Our North American friend, Canada, stipulates about 19 days off.

Recent research from the Pew Center found that 46 percent of US workers don't take all the time they are offered, presumably in lieu of making more money.[46] According to the *Harvard Business Review*, which cited a 2018 study, of about 768 million days of unused vacation time, 30 percent had been forfeited completely.[47]

Sadly, as a nation we are working ourselves to death. In Japan, they have a word for death from being overworked: *karoshi.*[48] They have a harsh working culture where overworked employees die from stress-related health conditions or suicide. The government attributes about 200 deaths per year to karoshi, but others estimate that number to be more like 10,000!

Studies have found workplace stress increases risk of heart attack and stroke.[49] If you are stressed half of the time at work, you are 25 percent more likely to suffer a fatal heart attack and have a 50 percent chance of dying of stroke. All work with no play really is dangerous! The adage is true: No one on their death bed ever wished that they could have one more day at work!

That is why it is so important not to miss the signs. First, don't ignore your stress, and don't self-medicate with unhealthy habits described in the section above, like drinking too much alcohol, using drugs, smoking, or overeating. If any of these accelerate, they may be signs to seek professional help. If you are feeling helpless and worthless and have thoughts of harming yourself, immediately call the U.S. Suicide and Crisis Lifeline: 988 (SMS also available). If you feel any signs of chest discomfort, have trouble breathing, neck, jaw or arm pain, indigestion, then you need to call 911 and visit the ER for a possible heart attack.

Next, you can take steps to reduce stress, like balancing your schedule with healthy activities, especially on your days off. Don't overcommit yourself, and try to plan regular breaks during your workday. You may need to prioritize your tasks, or break big work projects into smaller steps, and delegate responsibility whenever possible.

If you find yourself feeling resentful for working long hours, missing family time and events, and generally feeling unappreciated at work, these negative emotions will only add onto your stress.[50] Sometimes, the best thing to do is take a break, if you can, whether it is paid or not. As a physician, I do "prescribe" vacations. I tell my patients all the time that one of the best ways to take care of your physical and mental health is to take any time off and not think about work. Even a short weekend away[51] at regular intervals can do wonders!

The alternative cost of not taking vacations is too high! According to *Gallup Surveys*, workplace stress and employee engagement is a global, 8.8 trillion-dollar problem.[52] It estimated that it costs employers about up to $550 billion in lost productivity, $200 billion a year in absenteeism, as well as costs of staff turnover, workers compensation, and medical insurance. An average of 60 percent of lost workdays and productivity is related to stress.[53]

Employees under stress perform poorly at work; they make more mistakes, are more disorganized, have trouble concentrating, become frustrated and angry, and eventually stop caring and become burned out. The *Wall Street Journal* found about one-third of people consider quitting their job because of work stress and burnout.[54] Several surveys found that up to 40 percent of workers say they are extremely stressed-out at work.[55]

Vacations not only physically separate us from our day-to-day stresses, but also mentally separate us. There is some truth to the idiom that something "seems a million miles away." It's hard to sit on a beautiful beach and ruminate about paperwork or deadlines. That is why over three-quarters of respondents to a Nielsen Survey Research[56] reported feeling happier when they regularly vacationed. Periodic and regular vacations while taking time for yourself and your family lowers your stress level and decreases the release of all those stress hormones that contribute to degrading our mental and physical health.

The term *vacation sex* is a real phenomenon, especially for men who might have performance issues while worrying about work and financial pressures. And it's not all in their heads! Chronic stress and higher cortisol levels are associated with lower testosterone levels that contribute to loss of libido and interest in sex[57] as well as loss of energy and feeling depressed, which further adds to issues with libido.[58]

Taking a vacation is not selfish or extravagant. Instead, it's critical for your health to put yourself and your family first and regularly take some time to rest, relax, and recharge. It's a part of our life cycle of healthy choices. Think about the good feeling you get in anticipation of your upcoming vacation. Then think about how relaxed you actually feel while on your vacation. Being able to rest and recharge has been shown to improve performance and creativity at home and at work.[59] Many studies find that that vacation and leisure time can increase feelings of well-being,[60] and can improve family bonds.[61] To sum it up, you need to take a break because:

- Vacations are one of the best ways to relieve stress and actually increase productivity.
- Vacations can prevent burnout.
- Vacations actually keep us healthy by lowering levels of stress hormones like cortisol and epinephrine.
- Vacations promote an overall feeling of well-being.
- Vacations help with job performance, from psychological and physical benefits that have lasting effects on quality of life and work.
- Vacations are a gift to yourself, your partner, and your family!

Key Takeaways

- Don't sweat the small stuff. Doing so can jeopardize your health, so put yourself and your health first.
- Don't make retail therapy your go-to—debt and overspending will only increase your stress in the long run.
- Don't self-medicate. But don't beat yourself up about it either; it is not a character flaw, and there is professional help available.
- Don't diet. Restrictive diets are not maintainable and can cause harmful yo-yo dieting; instead, change your lifestyle choices slowly over time.
- Don't work yourself to death. Taking vacations or even a little time off of work benefits your physical and mental health and well-being, as well as your relationships at home and at work.

Chapter 8

Preparing and Handling Life's Inevitable Stresses

Life doesn't always play fair. As soon as we think life has settled down, stress seems to pop up around the corner. Some stress can be expected, while at other times, it comes out of nowhere. In this chapter, I want to address some stresses that we can actually see coming. They are inevitable, but we can be ready for them.

I'M NOT AGING GRACEFULLY!

Maybe it's the perfectionist in me, but I don't want to look bad, feel bad, or feel stressed with every birthday. I'd rather try to rewind my biological clock. And I hate to admit it, but I am willing to try just about anything. As the subtitle suggests, I am not aging gracefully; I am going—kicking and screaming!

Aging is one stress we can expect, but we don't have to give in to it completely either—and stress and aging are related.[1] Stress affects how we look and how we age, which is also interrelated with our overall health. My trademarked concept of "Health from the Outside In™" is about how the things we do that enhance our appearance on the outside can actually affect our health on the inside. I call it vanity's dirty little secret!

A Danish study corroborates that appearing older than your actual age is in fact an indicator of poor health.[2] Obviously, lifestyle factors like poor diet and lack of exercise, as well as smoking, wreak havoc on our health, but also our appearance. And not managing or trying to reduce your stress can have the same results.

Chronic stress affects facial appearance and accelerates the aging process. Research has shown chronic stress ages our skin.[3] Cortisol release increases inflammation and can break down collagen and elastin in our skin, causing wrinkles. Chronic stress can lead to insulin resistance, which can not only predispose us to diabetes, but higher blood sugars can also cause a metabolic process called glycation, which also negatively impacts skin elasticity.

Why do you think presidents seem to age so much while in office? It almost seems as if there are presidential years equivalent to dog years for those in office. Even on a cellular level, we age more during stress, causing cardiac dysfunction and immune dysfunction. In a study of women between the ages of 20 and 50, researchers found that the immune cells of those who lived with extreme stress (such as mothers who cared for their chronically ill children) tended to show signs of approximately 10 years worth of added aging, compared to those women who led less stressful lives.[4]

Even the idea of a bad hair day isn't a joke. According to a study conducted at Yale University,[5] bad hair days are real and the perception of having one produces negative consequences beyond not feeling good about how you look. It can affect your self-esteem and negatively impact your performance, causing stress and social anxiety. Researchers found that bad hair days increased self-doubt, intensified social insecurities, and resulted in more general self-criticism. Most notably, just the thought of having a bad hair day caused people to feel they weren't as smart as other people. People perceive their capabilities to be significantly lower than others when experiencing a bad hair day. Even though the study was funded through Proctor and Gamble, any woman on earth can attest to the results! And these findings were articulated by a serious psychology researcher at an Ivy League institution.

In fact, another study out of Stanford business school in the journal of *Organizational Behavior and Human Decision Processes* found similar results.[6] Researchers found that how we perceive our looks and our hair affects how we value ourselves and how we see ourselves in society. Feeling attractive can give us confidence and puts power into our hands.

Weight and body image can add to stress and decrease our self-esteem. A study looking at data from a variety of women and men found a clear relationship between body mass index (BMI) and body satisfaction, which also relates to happiness and positivity for overall well-being.[7] In this study, women tended to feel best about their bodies when their BMI was between 17.5 and 20. Women preferred being slightly underweight to low-end normal weight. Other studies have found that women can often have misperceptions about ideal body weight,[8] further driving a tendency to idealize underweight BMIs.

In fact, a study published in *Nature Scientific Reports* describes the established nervous system pathways that link self-esteem and our physical health.[9] The hippocampus, an area of the brain important in learning, memory, and emotional processing—including feelings of anxiety—also regulates another part of the brain, the hypothalamus-pituitary axis (HPA); the HPA acts as a link between our endocrine and nervous system, affecting many physical bodily functions, such as our autonomic nervous system, cardiovascular, metabolic, and immune systems. Therefore, feelings of inadequacy due to low self-esteem trigger our hippocampus and HPA axis, and over time, this stressful situation can age us.

We also know that there is a direct correlation between being overweight and numerous medical conditions, including high blood pressure, type 2 diabetes, and heart disease. There is also a direct correlation between weight and longevity: Thinner people tend to live longer than heavier people and tend to have fewer mobility issues. While I am not a proponent of having a number on the scale determine your happiness, despite my sometimes being a victim of this, there are no doubts about the benefits to maintaining a healthy weight and active lifestyle. And when you feel better about one thing, whether it's your hair or your weight or what you had for breakfast, you are more prone to do things that build on that feeling.

As stated in the prior chapter, there are dangers to rapidly and repeatedly losing and gaining weight, so called yo-yo dieting. Gaining and losing more than 11 pounds per year can make us look older, especially if we are over 50. Loss of facial fat can alter the architecture, increasing wrinkles and folds. Studies find that if we lose too much weight over the age of 50, we tend to look older than women of the same age who maintained a healthy amount of body fat.[10,11] Unfortunately, sometimes you have to choose whether you want a better-looking face or a smaller, perkier ass. It's a balancing act we all must work with as we age.

In fact, with the more widespread use of weight-loss drugs for treating obesity and diabetes, the first semaglutide brand name Ozempic, doctors have coined the term *Ozempic face*,[12] which describes a reduction in facial fat leading to sagging and wrinkles, but it can happen with any significant weight loss, regardless of method.

Let's take a closer look at wrinkles for a minute. Next to weight, they are a very prominent sign that you aren't taking care of yourself. They also make you look older than you are. Wrinkles aren't only due to genetics; they are also equally, maybe even more so, due to environmental factors, such as stress, abnormal weight gain and loss (the effects of yo-yo dieting), smoking, sun exposure, and eating the wrong kinds of food. So it's important to maintain a diet that is not only good for your heart but for your face too. People on a diet higher in fruits and vegetables and lower in animal fat tend to have less facial wrinkling and a more youthful appearance.[13,14]

In a study on wrinkles in identical twins, twins who suffered stressful situations, such as divorce, looked nearly two years older than their identical siblings who had not gone through a stressful situation.[15] Weight gain was another major factor in perceived age difference. In those sets of twins who were under 40 years of age, the heavier twin was perceived as being older, while in those who were over 40 years old, the heavier sibling appeared younger because, again, loss of too much weight as we age can age us. Most importantly, the presence of stress was a critical common denominator in those twins who appeared older in terms of wrinkles.

Some doctors have noted that people who start using antidepressants as soon as clinical depression is diagnosed tend to look much better and develop fewer lines as they age over people who waited to intervene in their depression. This stands to reason, since doctors know that when people are depressed, there is a tendency to neglect self-care. Coupled with a tendency to perhaps drink or eat more, as a way of self-medicating, or maybe take up or increase smoking, neglect takes on a dangerous and unflattering life of its own. When people are happier, including depressed people who identify and take an effective antidepressant, they find healthy ways to reduce stress, and they tend to look younger. And studies corroborate this; antidepressants can lower your cortisol levels.[16] Antidepressants have anti-inflammatory properties too.[17] And chronic inflammation, which can lead to metabolic syndrome and diabetes as well as heart disease, also takes a toll on your skin, a concept called *inflamm-aging*.[18,19]

But the good news is that we can take charge to help prevent this inevitable stress. Healthy lifestyle decisions, as well as a positive attitude, can help to prevent premature aging. I hope I've convinced you that vanity can be a healthy motivator to fight off the stress of aging. It can be a virtue when it comes to your health. Once you decide that you're worth it (and you are!), and you start getting selfish about taking time to care for yourself, you've made great progress.

The first step in enjoying the benefits of vanity is to try to change your attitude and focus on reducing the stress in your life. If you even just pretend to care about the way you look and go through the motions of grooming and healthy living, it can have a real impact. Eventually, you will start to believe in it, and it will become a way of life that may even become second nature. I wrote about just that in a blog on my website years ago.

Back Away from the Yoga Pants!
By Leigh Vinocur MD

So far, it's been one month, and I have been keeping my one and only New Year's resolution and that has automatically kept me on track with my weight, exercise, and getting organized. This is my New Year mantra: Back away from the yoga pants . . . all day!

Yoga pants and workout clothes have become a fashion staple for many women, me included. So many big designers and even celebrities have their own workout lines such as Beyonce, Carrie Underwood, Kate Hudson, and Heidi Klum, just to name a few.

In fact, the fashion industry makes them so cute, in a huge assortment of matching colors and styles and price points, that they are irresistible. It takes no effort or thought process to pick out a cute outfit. They are like those old mix-and-match pajama sets for kids called Garanimals; but for adults, you can instantly mix and match that perfect outfit, with no decisions! And I don't have to tell you about the comfort! You could practically sleep in them. So, you may ask, why my New Year boycott? It's actually the ease and comfort that poses the "danger!"

It creates a domino effect. These comfy, ready-made outfits allowed me to get out the door in minutes. No hair, no makeup, they are the perfect complement to some sunscreen (I never leave home without it) and a baseball cap. Perfect for the busy working mom.

But my nana would have been horrified! She would never leave the house without at least foundation, rouge, lipstick, and her hair done up, although it was her 60's hair-sprayed helmet-do. I thought that was ridiculous; you're a slave to other people's perception? I am an intelligent, educated woman. I don't care what people think about the way I look. I am liberated and I don't need makeup to go out. But what I have slowly discovered over time is that maybe Nana was on to something.

At work, I often wear baggy scrubs; it's hard to be glamorous as an ER doc if you're splashed with vomit, poop, and blood! I'd be so tired after shifts on my days off that it was just easier to run around with unwashed hair and stretchy workout clothes. But it made me feel sloppy, despite the cute, coordinated outfits. And the sloppier I felt, the worse I felt about myself. I seemed to get sloppier at home, too. The more my home got disorganized, the more I felt like eating. And those stretchy, soft, and comfy yoga pants were very accommodating for those extra pounds that began to sneak up on me! And the more I ate, the less I actually felt like working out, which is both counterintuitive and ironic for a broad running around in workout clothes all the time! It would seem that my bad hair was making me feel down.

There really is some science behind a bad hair day. A Yale Study found that bad hair days could affect a person's self-esteem by increasing their self-doubt and making them more insecure and self-critical to the point that they perceive their own capabilities as lower than others!

That is exactly what happened to me. It was a vicious cycle of not caring what I looked like and starting to feel worse and worse. Thus, my single New Year's resolution was no more yoga pants! Even if it does take a little extra effort, I feel better already. I am organizing my house again, eating healthier, and getting up earlier to work out—in my yoga pants, of course! But that's it, off they come when I shower and change.

Sure, I know it's okay to run out with my baseball cap, workout gear, and just sunscreen when I really need to or feel like it; however, I've found some liberation in a little lipstick, mascara and a blowout, and the point is that I am doing it for me. I still don't care what other people think, but I care what I think I look like. I am putting that extra effort into myself; to say yes, I am worth it! And it's been paying off. Thanks, Nana ;-)

Originally Published on drleigh.com

WHEN IT'S MORE THAN A BAD HAIR DAY

I don't want to trivialize the importance of diagnosing clinical depression. If stress, anxiety, and sadness are getting in the way of taking care of yourself, you may need professional guidance or an intervention. The classic symptoms of depression include:[20]

- Having little interest or pleasure in doing things
- Feeling down or hopeless
- Lethargy but difficulty falling asleep or staying asleep
- Inability to concentrate
- Decreased appetite for a sustained period of time
- Feeling bad about yourself consistently over a long period of time
- Feeling like loved ones and the world would be better off without you
- Thoughts of hurting yourself and/or suicidal ideation

It may seem like these signs would be easy to detect, but I have met patients who just complain of various aches and pains when they are really struggling with regulating their mood. You simply may not realize what's going on, but you know that something's not right. That means it's crucial that you talk to your doctor. Don't be afraid to tell your doctor that you feel off, even if you can't pinpoint specific reasons why. Your doctor can ask you a series of questions that should help you determine if you're seriously depressed or not. Not all depression is permanent, and the treatment could be seeing a mental health professional for counseling and talk therapy, or pharmaceutical therapy. It's important to act on your depression, because living with depression not only affects your mental health, it can also affect your physical health and put your life at risk.

Adult females with clinical depression are 29 percent more likely to suffer a stroke than women of the same age without depression, according to Harvard researchers.[21] American Heart Association published data that depression can worsen heart disease[22] or even cause it in younger people.[23] Depression is a serious matter. Aside from its negative impact on your health, it can cause people to take drastic measures. I am talking about suicide; while most depressed patients don't attempt suicide it's always a risk.[24] Many people dance around the issue and are afraid to bring it up with loved ones, but it is critical to ask someone if they are considering it. It is also important to let them know that they are not alone.

Now, it is easier than ever to get help because a new national hotline for suicide prevention just went into effect. Instead of having to remember or look up a 10-digit phone number, the new Suicide and Crisis Lifeline is just three numbers: 988.[25]

AVOID BECOMING A HEART DISEASE OR CANCER STATISTIC

Heart disease and cancer are the top two leading causes of death for women in the US. Most women don't realize that, despite the American Heart Association's National Go Red for Women campaign, which was started in 2004 to bring heart disease awareness to women.[26] According to the CDC, still only about half of women realize that heart disease is their greatest health risk.[27] It's our number one killer! This gender bias can also be seen in physicians who are less likely to diagnosis heart disease in middle-age women.[28]

As mentioned earlier in the book, this is not so if you are seen by a female doctor in the ER! I'm proud to say that a study found that women coming into the ER with a heart attack who were treated by women emergency physicians were less likely to die.[29] And it isn't only in the ER that we see benefits. The *Journal of the American Medical Association-Internal Medicine* published study that found that patients were more likely to survive a hospitalization and not be readmitted if they were treated by female physicians.[30]

I am proud to say that women physicians tend to listen more; they are more communicative and spend more time with patients.[31] They tend stick to clinical guidelines more.[32] They also tend to take more time counseling patients on preventative care.[33] So let's hear it for the girls!

Unfortunately, our exemplary care is not rewarded, as there is still a huge gender pay gap for women physicians; on average, we make $20,000 less![34] But that is a topic for another book, even though it is another stress-inducing factor that we women must manage!

Another health tragedy is that almost half of cancer deaths are either completely preventable or detectable at such an early stage that they are curable, according to the American Cancer Society[35] and other studies.[36]

For these reasons alone, women should be crystal clear about our top two enemies and know how to avoid them. By taking a few steps, we don't have to become a statistic, and we'll be healthier with less stress and, obviously, look much better too.

THE UGLY TRUTH ABOUT HEART
DISEASE FOR WOMEN

- In the US, cardiovascular disease kills more women than all forms of cancer combined.[37]
- 42 percent of women die within one year of a heart attack compared with only 24 percent of men.[38]
- Risk factors like diabetes, smoking, and high cholesterol can negate any cardiovascular protection estrogen confers to younger women.[39]
- Women who smoke have their heart attacks 19 years earlier than non-smokers.[40]
- Two-thirds of women who die suddenly from heart disease had no prior symptoms or history.[41]
- Women who have heart attacks under the age of 50 are twice as likely to die from them as men.[42]

HEART MATTERS

Why do women die more often than men due to heart disease? Several reasons, but on top of the list is that we are second-class citizens when it comes to heart disease; women are not diagnosed with heart-related conditions as quickly as men. Studies show that when they present to the emergency room with chest pain, it is often underestimated and assumed not to be cardiac in nature.[43] We are also not treated with recommended medications and procedures as often as men.[44] Perhaps that's why, when heart disease is finally diagnosed and treated, we don't fare as well.

According to the American Heart Association (AHA), cardiovascular disease kills more women than men every year, and almost 10 times more women than breast cancer.[45] So where is the advocacy, the indignation, the walks for a cure? It's possible that because breast cancer, with its outward visible scars, is still more jarring for women than heart disease, which is ten times more deadly.

Some of the blame lies with us. We are notorious for putting our own health last. We are vigilant when it comes to the health of our spouses and children. Women are often the gatekeepers of health for the whole family. We go to appointments and ask questions; however, no one does the same for us. I have seen very few men accompany their wives to medical appointments with documented internet research and a list of questions the way women do for their husbands. But by taking care of ourselves we are, in fact, benefiting the whole family.

It isn't always that women blatantly ignore their symptoms; many women don't even realize they are having symptoms of a heart attack. There are significant gender differences between the recognizable symptoms.[46] For example, unlike men who have easily identifiable crushing chest pain and shortness of breath (see Gender Difference in Symptoms of Heart Attack), many women have vague complaints that could easily be attributed to other problems such as nausea, sweating, indigestion, or fatigue.

Gender Difference in Symptoms of Heart Attack

Men

- Crushing chest pain or pressure (described as an elephant on your chest)
- Sweating
- Shortness of breath
- Pain in arms, neck, or jaw

Women

- Indigestion
- Unusual fatigue
- Anxiety, sweating
- Possibly chest pain
- Jaw, shoulder or arm pain
- Shortness of breath
- Change in sleeping pattern

We need to know our symptoms but, more importantly, we need to know our risk factors,[47] such as smoking and a strong family history or diabetes. And we need to know our numbers for blood pressure, cholesterol, and waist circumference. A larger waist circumference puts us at risk for diabetes and heart disease.[48] One or more risks can totally negate any beneficial protection estrogen gives to younger women with respect to heart disease. Historically it's that idea of the estrogen benefit that might have initially created the bias we see in medicine today. Prevention is the best intervention! We need to empower ourselves and take action. The more we pay attention to our own heart health, the more we will get our doctors to do the same. And don't take no for an answer; if you feel you're still having a problem, don't stop until you find a doctor who listens to you and finds the problem. And as we discussed in the prior chapters—maybe it should be a woman cardiologist!

THE "BIG C"

I am not talking about Vitamin C here. I am talking about the word that evokes fear with every mention: *cancer*. Cancer is the second leading cause of death among women in the US and can attack just about every organ in the body. Back in 1987, lung cancer was the leading cause of cancer death in US women, surpassing breast cancer.[49]

Lung cancer is the leading cause of cancer deaths in this country for both men and women, with 87 percent due to tobacco—whether smoked or chewed.[50] Tobacco accounts for more than lung cancer, with 30 percent of deaths coming from cancer in the mouth, nasal cavity, larynx, pharynx, esophagus, also stomach, liver, pancreas, kidney, bladder, and cervix, to name a few! Unfortunately, 80 percent of smokers started before they were 18 years old, so the better we can encourage our kids to stay away from smoking, the better.

The number one thing you can do to prevent this cancer is *quit smoking*! I know it's addicting, and it's hard to break bad habits, but keep trying. Talk to your doctor and ask for prescription drugs that can be used in combination with over-the-counter gums and patches.

Lifestyle factors, such as eating nutritious foods, exercising regularly, and maintaining a healthy weight, help reduce your risk of developing cancer.[51] But still, the earlier you can detect any cancer, the better the prognosis. And for many, early detection can make them curable.

Here are just a few key cancer screening guidelines, but you should always discuss these with your doctor; they should be individualized according to your medical history. Women, especially those who are sexually active in their 20s, should begin annual pap smear exams to identify cervical cancer, as well as HPV testing. There are also now vaccines against HPV, sometimes given to teens girls and young adults that can prevent the strains of HPV known to cause cervical cancer, as well as certain mouth, head, and neck cancers.[52]

Unfortunately, even well before the vaccine mistrust that came with the COVID-19 pandemic, there was an issue back when this HPV vaccine became available. I wrote an article on this topic in 2010.

HPV Vaccine: Why Are So Few People Getting Vaccinated?
By Leigh Vinocur, MD

An alarming new study from the University of Maryland School of Medicine finds, sadly, very few young women are protecting themselves from cancer and getting the HPV vaccine.

It is probably one of the most significant medical breakthroughs of this past decade. A vaccine to prevent cancer! We now better understand the link between cancers and viruses and how some viruses, such as the human papillomavirus (HPV), can change cells and cause them to become cancerous. In essence, we have identified a communicable form of cancer.

HPV is often a sexually transmitted disease, which, according to the Centers for Disease Control and Prevention (CDC), is very common and infects about 6 million people a year. It's estimated that 50 percent of sexually active men and women have been exposed to it at some point in their lives. There are hundreds of strains of HPV; about 30 to 40 of the strains are sexually transmitted. In the majority of infections, the immune system takes care of it without any treatment. However, some of these sexually transmitted infections can cause cervical cancer. It's the high-risk strains of the virus that remain in the body and cause a long-term infection. It then invades the cells of the cervix, causing changes in the cellular structure and DNA to become pre-cancerous lesions as well as cause genital warts. If these infections aren't detected and treated, they can eventually go on to become an invasive cervical cancer.

The National Cancer Institute estimates that 12,200 women in the United States will be diagnosed with this type of cancer and nearly 4,200 women will die from it. Worldwide cervical cancer strikes nearly half a million women each year, killing almost 250,000.

But we now have developed a monumental vaccine that protects against the common HPV strains that cause about 70 percent of cervical cancers. HPV has also been recently linked to 26 percent of head and neck cancers, as well as some vulvar, vaginal, penile, and rectal cancers. This discovery has opened a new door for prevention of cancer.

Yet, an alarming new study from the University of Maryland School of Medicine finds sadly very few young women are protecting themselves from cancer and taking this precaution of the HPV vaccine. This study led by Dr. J. Kathleen Tracy found that less than 30 percent of young women eligible for the vaccine will choose to get it. Added to that, of the women who do initiate getting vaccinated, less than one-third complete the series of three booster shots required for full protection from the virus. Young African American women were the least likely to complete the series of shots.

The CDC currently recommends beginning vaccination of girls 11 to 12 years of age with completion of a series of 3 shots up to age 26. The hope is to vaccinate young women before they become very sexually active and become exposed to the virus.

There is a debate among scientists on whether adolescent boys should also be vaccinated. While men don't have cervical cancer, they do get genital warts, head and neck, as well as penile and rectal cancers. Recent research has shown a new demographic of younger men with head and neck cancers that never smoked or drank alcohol, which was considered a risk factor in these cancers. Instead, these younger demographics of patients were found to be HPV-positive.

So, the same way the virus gets into cells of the cervix and changes the cells, it does the same with the cells in the mouth and throat.

The public health community also advocates vaccination of boys as a form of herd immunity. What this means is that if we vaccinate boys, we will see less men walking around with HPV, and thus fewer women will be infected. However, the CDC came in just short of a recommendation for boys, stating physicians and parents have the option to vaccinate them. But this University of Maryland study shows we are not even vaccinating our daughters. It is disturbing for me as a physician and a mother to see a safe and effective vaccine that can protect against cancer be so underutilized!

Perhaps it is suggestive of our collective lack of emphasis on preventive medicine as a whole. Our sedentary lifestyle and obesity rate is a testament to that. We are so good in the American medical community at fixing and treating chronic diseases after they happen; we need to now concentrate on providing more preventive measures for our patients, as well as emphasizing to them that they must bear some personal responsibility to maintain their health with good habits.

Add to the mix our misguided distrust of all vaccines. We seem to have short-term memory when it comes to the tens of thousands of children that died every year not long ago from infectious diseases that we now give immunizations for and take for granted. Now, unless vaccines are mandated for things such as school enrollment, we don't bother, as evidenced by our yearly battle with the flu vaccine.

Or perhaps it's our prudish mores, which don't approve of vaccines that protect us from sexually transmitted infections. Some groups feel it might in some way be sending the wrong message to young girls. Certainly no one in the medical community is advocating sexually promiscuity for young women, nor trying to send the message that safe sex is no longer needed once you are vaccinated. We are also continuing to advocate pap smear exams for women at the age of 21 or for those who are sexually active.

But whatever the reasons, this vaccination rate is a travesty. We as parents want to protect our children from everything and years ago, if someone had told you they had a shot to prevent cancer, it would seem like a miracle. It makes no sense now; with all our earnest endeavors and talk of trying to find a cure for cancer, we are overlooking our children's chances to prevent it in the first place.

Originally Published on HuffingtonPost.com

Another exam to consider in your 20s is a skin exam; both a self-exam of all your dark spots and moles to look for any changes over time and a yearly dermatologist evaluation can help detect, early, one of the deadliest skin cancers: melanoma.

Even though the United States Preventive Services Taskforce (USPSTF) recommends annual mammograms starting at age 50,[53] they are very conservative, and most women end up having have at least one mammogram by their mid-40s, in addition to monthly self-breast exams. But obviously if you have a family history with a first-degree relative who had breast cancer, you and your doctor may opt to begin earlier.

For colon and rectal cancer, the USPSTF recommends beginning colonoscopy at 50, but recently, we have seen a rise in colorectal cancer in younger people—even without risk factors such as family history or inflammatory bowel diseases such as Crohn's or ulcerative colitis. Most physicians have now moved colonoscopy screening up to the mid-40s, but again, even earlier with risk factors and a discussion with your doctor. These are just some general guidelines; they will vary based on your risk factors, family history, and lifestyle. So check with your doctor about when you should begin screening and how often you should be screened.

While there is still a debate as to whether healthy people without symptoms need a yearly comprehensive physical,[54] that is probably more driven by economics and insurance companies. There is research that shows the public wants these yearly exams.[55] And since the passage of the Affordable Care Act in 2010, preventative care and exams had to be included with private insurers.[56]

THE ALMIGHTY MAMMARY

Let's delve into breast cancer a bit more, because despite heart disease being women's number one killer, more women worry about breast cancer.[57] Breasts are one way to define the mammal class in the animal kingdom. These mammary glands distinguish us from other animals because we nurse and nurture our young, but no other mammal comes close to how humans have objectified, sexualized, and idolized the almighty mammary glands.

Whatever you call them—boobs, tits, ta-tas, or cans—we humans are obsessed with breasts. And it is not just men; many women are obsessed about their shape, firmness, and size. Many of us let our breasts define us.

The art world has glorified breasts in sculptures and paintings. Hollywood reveres them. The fashion industry celebrates and decorates them, with padded, pushed up, revealing, low-cut décolletage and cleavage-bearing styles. Perhaps our attachment to our breasts comes from the fact that our mothers did nurture us with them. Therefore, it makes the ironic twist even crueler that an organ, which at one time literally sustained life, can turn so sinister in the cancerous state.

Breast cancer is one of the most emotional diseases for women. It invokes literal armies of advocates trying to defeat it, even though heart disease is our number one health threat. It may seem counterintuitive, but even when it comes to breast cancer treatment, the saying may stand: Less is actually more!

A study published in *Cancer* found that women who had early-stage breast cancer had better survival rates if they had lumpectomy and radiation, as opposed to total mastectomy.[58] Prior studies[59] have shown that in tumors up to 5 centimeters (less than 2 inches) in size, lumpectomy and radiation is just as effective as mastectomy for long-term survival. So there's hope for saving your breasts, based on this large, real-life study that shows that we don't have to default to having a mastectomy.

Lumpectomy is the surgical removal of the breast tumor with a surrounding rim of healthy tissue. It must be combined with radiation of that same breast to ensure no cancer is left behind. It is also called breast-conserving surgery. It cannot be performed if the tumor is too large, if there is more than one tumor in the breast, or if for any other reason a person may not be able to have the required coinciding radiation, such as in pregnancy.

Breast-conserving surgery was first described back in the late '70s as an answer to the radical and disfiguring older technique of mastectomy, called the Halsted radical mastectomy. This procedure was named after the surgeon who developed it back in 1894. It involved removing the whole breast, all the lymph nodes under the arm with its surrounding tissue and underlying muscles, leaving what little skin was left to be stretched across the rib cage. This type of surgery was a common treatment for breast cancer for more than 75 years.

My grandmother had the procedure in the '60s and never let my mom see her bare-chested again; she claimed it was too horrible to see. The procedure left women with trouble using their arms because of the muscle removed. The molecular science we now know about how breast cancer develops and spreads has shown us that there is no need for such a radical measure. While no surgeons are doing Halstead's radical surgery anymore,[60] even today younger women are opting for mastectomies over breast conserving therapies.

The likely reason behind this is there is still such fear associated with the Big C. Psychologically, women just want it out of their bodies. And who can blame them? Despite what I know scientifically as a physician, as a patient, I think I would feel the same way! It is a very frightening decision women must make. In fact, when my beloved mother was diagnosed over 30 years ago, I was in my surgical residency, and I begged her to have a mastectomy because I was petrified of losing her. She refused.

Maybe it was her experience with her mom's Halsted, but looking back at what she said made sense. She told me that if it were going to recur, she would rather have the cancer come back in that same breast than in her chest wall, which was closer to her lungs. Her breast cancer never did come back.

Radiation is only used to treat local disease in that surrounding breast after lumpectomy. It kills any potential cancer cells left behind after a lumpectomy. It is not used after a mastectomy, and surgeons don't have microscopic vision while doing surgery. So even if a surgeon has a pathologist check the margins during the mastectomy to try to remove all the cancer, it only takes one cell left behind to start to grow again.

Breast cancer still evokes a primal, visceral fear in women. How can an organ, that literally nurtures and sustains life and is the object of beauty and pleasure, turn deadly? Often, for those of us who are faced with this disease, it's hard to do less. It feels like we must take charge and go to battle with all we have! Fortunately, we continue to see new research every year with different treatment options, new drugs, new surgery techniques, new types of radiation therapies as part of our armamentarium, which will help us become more informed to make these very difficult and personal decisions with our physicians.

THE M-WORD

I don't mean money, which can be another source of stress that we've already discussed. I am talking about menopause. It is a rite of passage, a natural biological process marking the end of a woman's reproductive years, typically occurring between the ages of 45 and 55. It is defined by the cessation of menstruation for twelve consecutive months, indicative of the ovaries no longer releasing eggs. Menopause affects millions of women worldwide and is accompanied by various physiological and psychological changes that can significantly impact quality of life.

Sometimes it is known by a host of amusing names,[61] most commonly the change. But there are others—some I had not known before my research for this book, such as ovarian retirement, internal furnace, super-soaker event, reverse puberty, private summer, power surges, nightcrawlers, brain fog, and closed baby factory, just to name a few! Many are self-explanatory from the symptoms we have, but the Chinese, whose culture tends to revere old age and its wisdom more than we do, have a name that translates to "second spring."[62]

Traditionally, spring signals a new beginning, but this is a second beginning—for a new phase of life. It really sounds lovely until you start to feel the itching from the dry skin; the painful sex from vaginal dryness; the bitching, irritability, and crying from the crazy mood swings and those damn hot flashes and night sweats. Then it does not seem so pastoral and pretty! Many of these symptoms can start four to eight years before actual menopause; it's called perimenopause.[63]

It is a long, sometimes awful transition from our waning reproductive years to menopause, and our hormone—estrogen, estradiol, and progesterone—levels can fluctuate the whole time. We know how this roller coaster of changing hormone levels affect both our physical and emotional health.[64] Unfortunately, there is not a big curriculum devoted to this topic in med school. Even for those medical school graduates who go on to OB/GYN residencies, studies[65] show that only about one-third of OB/GYN residency programs have a curriculum on menopause! It is unbelievable to me that these women's health specialists and experts are not even getting enough training!

Many women feel invisible after menopause, or they want to be invisible while losing the hair on their head as the hair on their chins and upper lips grows or the weight gain piles on the mid-section—pot bellies, some call it menopot. It's terrible. That is why I call estrogen the wonder drug! I miss my estrogen. And in fact, during the follicular phase,[66] the estrogen part of our menstrual cycle, our maturing follicles prepare for ovulation and our estradiol levels are high and we feel more energized, more creative, and happier! That is because serotonin, a brain neurochemical that elevates our mood, increases during that time and there is a link.[67]

The impending release of our egg during ovulation, which evolutionarily makes sense for propagation of our species, is the time when we feel more desirable and attractive.[68] By the way, the next phase of menstruation, called the luteal phase, occurs after the egg is ovulated and the follicles produce progesterone; during this time, we can feel a bit crappy with bloating, fluid retention, and fatigue—what we think of as PMS. This can also correspond to rises in our stress hormone, cortisol, contributing to these symptoms, and even anxiety and depression.[69] Therefore, it is no wonder that once menopause occurs, without much estrogen circulation, we naturally feel terrible.

This topic is, of course, big enough for a series of books, so I can only address some general issues on how to deal with this as one of the inevitable life stressors that we will all eventually face.

AM I GOING CRAZY?

Let's start with your emotions, and no, you are not going crazy or getting dementia. Many of us experience laughing one minute and crying the next— over seemingly nothing; it can feel like puberty's moody cousin has come to visit us. And the forgetfulness—never being able to find our keys, phones, or reading glasses—is maddening! Some studies have found that 60 percent of women have these memory lapses.[70]

This brain fog[71] often goes away on its own when hormone levels stabilize a bit, but it can also be associated with anxiety related to our changing physiological systems. Just like with any stress or anxiety problems, lifestyle changes such as exercise, healthy eating, and sleep are important, but if severe anxiety occurs, make sure you speak with a mental health professional. And likewise, a little forgetfulness, such as misplacing your keys, is common for everyone, menopause or not. But if you find them and don't know what they are used for, well, that is another issue completely, and you definitely need to talk to a physician.

NATURE'S PRANK: HOT FLASHES AND THE NOSTALGIA FOR DRY SHEETS

Now, I do realize that the recommendation of getting enough sleep sounds ridiculous, especially because the hot flashes (vasomotor symptoms) and night sweats (the biggest complaint related to menopause) that wake you up in the middle of the night with soaking-wet sheets. This messed-up, unpredictable internal thermostat makes you feel like you are wearing a fur coat in the Sahara Desert. Jokes aside, they can seriously affect your quality of life and cause sleep problems. That's probably why they are the main reason many women seek hormone replacement therapy (HRT).

THE COMPLICATED HISTORY OF HORMONE REPLACEMENT THERAPY (HRT)

The history of HRT is very complex and somewhat controversial. Menopause, although completely natural, has been medicalized[72] and called hormone deficiency syndrome, because men did not want to hear about women's issues. Back in the 1800s,[73] ovarian cow tissue was implanted in women, and it wasn't until late in that century that doctors started to understand the importance of antiseptic medical practices.[74] I imagine, like a lot of medicine back then, the cure could be worse than the "disease."

It was around 1941[75] that estrogen was isolated from the urine of pregnant horses, called Premarin (from pregnant mares), and the medical community pushed to treat all women as a way to "maintain their femininity." By 1975, Premarin was the fifth most commonly prescribed drug in the US.[76] But what the medical community found out was that if you still had your uterus, the unopposed constant flow of estrogen caused uterine endometrial cancer,[77] so women had to also take a progesterone medication—essentially causing them to continue to menstruate past the reproductive age. Women accepted this because the medical community said it could also help with osteoporosis and heart disease.

But in the 1990s, the Women's Health Initiative (WHI), one of the largest clinical trials on women's health, was started; the part that specifically looked at heart disease was called the Heart Estrogen/Progestin Replacement Study (HERS)[78] and they found that hormone replacement therapy (HRT) did not help with heart disease. In fact, there was an increased risk of heart attack, stroke, pulmonary embolism (blood clot in the lungs), and breast cancer. Many women in the trial did smoke, and we know that smoking puts you at risk for heart attacks and blood clots, even in younger women who are just on oral birth control hormones, but after these studies, HRT was maligned and no longer recommended at all.

Even in medicine, extremes are not helpful, and moderation is key. Current research and thinking are that short-term use, about three to seven years of HRT for things like hot flashes for which it has the most benefit, is probably safe depending on your personal health risks and your family history;[79,80] but it is a personal choice you must make with your doctor.

There are newer non-hormonal drugs[81] on the market that just deal with hot flashes, also called vasomotor symptoms, but because they are new, like with any new medication, we don't yet know the long-term effects. There are also many supplements touted for helping with hot flashes, such as black cohosh,[82] or phytoestrogens such as soy,[83] but there can be drug interactions and making sure you have a high-quality supplement—verified by a third party that tests it to ensure purity, potency, and no contaminations with mold or bacteria—is key.

Bioidentical hormones have been gaining some popularity. They are compounded in special pharmacies, but they can have the same risks[84] and side effects as regular HRT. So again, it is important to discuss with your health-care provider. As far as heart-disease risk, like we discussed previously, lifestyle factors are key to reducing your risk.

NO BONES ABOUT IT

While it is true that HRT can help with osteoporosis, you must, again, weigh the risks. Modify your lifestyle, ensuring you get enough calcium and vitamin D and weight-bearing exercises. There are a host of non-hormonal treatments, as well, called bisphosphonates; talk with your doctor to help you make informed decisions.[85]

SEX IN THE SAND

That is the way most women describe sex after menopause due to vaginal dryness. I remember being at a dinner party not too long ago with a crowd of all the women there around me talking and asking questions about this. When my husband asked what we were all discussing and I told him it was vaginal dryness, he said, "Sorry I asked!"

But it is so true, and many women feel they don't have anyone to discuss this with, but you should be able to talk to your gynecologist about this. Lubricants alone often do not help because beyond the dryness, there is atrophy of the delicate tissues of the labia and opening of the vagina.[86] This atrophy can cause tears and pain during intercourse, so you need to do more than lubricate; that is why topical estrogen local only to the area can be a miracle cure! Because it only absorbs into the local tissues, there is none of the other risks seen with systemic estrogen, such as oral pills or patches or gels. In fact, even breast cancer survivors can use it without increased risk.[87]

Here is the trick that many doctors don't tell you when you get your prescription: It comes with a dispenser to inject cream inside the vagina. But guess what? That is not where the problem is for painful sex. You need to take just a tiny bit and rub it like hand cream around your inside labia and the opening of the vagina. After a couple of weeks, you will notice better stretching of the areas without any pain, and sex will not be painful either! Now you are ready to take advantage and enjoy postmenopausal sex, which can be very liberating. There are no more worries about pregnancy, so you can now have a more spontaneous and enjoyable sex life!

While menopause can bring its share of challenges, it's also a time of great freedom and a chance to focus more on yourself. Many women do report feeling more confident and less constrained by societal expectations as they age.

TURN HOLIDAY STRESS INTO SUCCESS

Holidays are other inevitable events in our lives. There always seems to be a holiday around the corner that makes us feel unprepared. And while they do bring loads of family, food, and fun, they can also be *stressful*!

Holidays can bring out the best and the worst in us. They can bring up memories of those we've lost, bring up pressures to put on a smiley face while dealing with the brokenness or dysfunction in our families. There are so many ways that holidays can be more stressful than restful. If you're secretly dreading the holidays, you're not alone! With more to do and less time to do it, holiday stress can get magnified ten times over. But never fear, I've got ideas to make you cheer.

One way to change holiday stress into success is to forget the big family gathering at your house and take a vacation! We all love vacations, so why not a holiday vacation? If your house is the place where the family gathering always happens, then you know that all the planning, communication, decorations, gifts, meals, and basically everything falls on you! Despite the extra helping hands at your home, you often end up with too many relatives staying over, giving you no time or space to relax. Plus, you wind up with all the chores during that time, too, such as laundry, cooking, and cleaning.

So, imagine the family packing their bags and taking a cruise where someone else does the cooking and cleaning! There are all-inclusive resorts, or meet-ups in the mountains near a ski resort, or other getaway spot! Let everyone know that instead of exchanging gifts, their gift to you and other loved ones is showing up at this large family vacation; make the experience the gift, while making great memories in the process. This lets everyone, including you, relax and enjoy each other's company while doing something different.

A recent travel survey by the AARP[88] showed that 98 percent of multi-generational travelers are highly satisfied taking trips with parents, kids, and grandparents. Besides, this way you will actually get to spend time with your family, instead of listening to their conversations through the kitchen door!

Along those same lines, if shopping for gifts during the holidays is stressful, then don't shop for things; instead, shop for experiences! When Cyber Monday rolls around, if you find yourself spending more money on stuff than you should, you are not alone. Think about it, does your son really need another video game to keep him on the couch? Does your daughter need another pair of boots? What if you could give your family something that will stay with them for life? A priceless memory from a shared experience. As corny as that may sound, studies[89] have found that experiential purchases, money spent on doing something, usually together as a family, tend to provide more enduring happiness than material purchases. Let your imagination run with this. How about a hot-air balloon ride, horseback camping trip, or tickets to the US Open Tennis Championships or to a concert? Whatever you think of, that you know your spouse or kids enjoy, you're sure to gift a forever-memory instead of another sweater stuffed away in the closet.

WHAT TO EXPECT WHEN YOU'RE NOT EXPECTING...IN THE ER

Another inevitable life stress and often a frightening experience is ending up in the ER. Sometimes, we can defeat stress by knowing what to expect. Because none of us expects to be there. But you can prepare yourself for the next time you're not expecting it.

Emergency rooms can be very scary places. With the fear of the unknown in a medical emergency, it's no surprise most people want to avoid the ER like the plague. With over 155 million[90] people, about 45 percent of our population, being treated in ERs every year, it is one of those inevitable stresses we will probably have to deal with at one time or another. What follows are a few facts and typical questions people have when in the ER. Understanding this may help balance your stress levels about the ER experience, and help you focus on what matters: you or your loved one's health and recovery.

WHY ERS ARE SO DARN CROWDED?

I'm with you. We emergency docs have been screaming about the system being overtaxed for years! Still, we need to accept the fact that emergency medical care is the safety net for our whole healthcare system. It's often the first place we visit after an emergency, because we can't waltz into our primary physician's office with an emergency.

This safety net is provided for everyone, regardless of their ability to pay. That's thanks to the Emergency Medical Treatment and Labor Act (EMTALA), a federal law that assures everyone's equal right to emergency care. Since the federal government mandates EMTALA, the emergency departments must care for all emergency cases that come in to the ER.

Before the Affordable Care Act, there were a lot of uninsured and underinsured patients, which resulted in uncompensated care, causing hospitals to become insolvent—and many closed. This is especially true in rural America.[91] Today, even with more insured patients, there are still fewer emergency and hospital beds, combined with down-sided nursing staff and on-call specialists seeing emergency patients, this all leads to boarding patients overnight in the ER, which can impact everyone's access to care.[92] This leads to ambulance diversions, a backlog in the waiting rooms, and gridlock of the system. This domino effect contributes to the dangerous overcrowding.

This is why during any cold, flu, or viral outbreak—the pandemic especially—many ERs became crippled. My cautionary tale is not intended to scare you away, but to give you an understanding of what ER nurses and doctors face every day. Still, it may surprise you that emergency medicine in the US is one of the most advanced systems in the world, and our ERs save countless lives every day regardless of these challenging circumstances.

Considering ER doctors, nurses, and other staff are barraged with a wide variety of cases and severity, we are capable of handling just about anything thrown at us.

The recent advent of urgent care centers has not fully decompressed the system for true emergencies.[93] There is the added fact that this is called retail medicine, and there is no federal mandate to see everyone regardless of their ability to pay, the way it is in the emergency department. And while they do serve a purpose, here's a quick guide on what is a true emergency that should be seen in the ER, how an emergency department really functions, and what's in store for you when you're there.

WHAT IS A TRUE EMERGENCY?

According to the American College of Emergency Physicians, these are the critical warning signs or symptoms[94] of a true emergency, and what any prudent layperson[95] could reasonably identify as an emergency.

1) Difficulty breathing, shortness of breath
2) Chest or upper abdominal pain or pressure
3) Fainting, sudden dizziness or weakness
4) Sudden change in vision
5) Confusion or changes in levels of consciousness (called mental status)
6) Any sudden severe pain
7) Uncontrolled bleeding
8) Severe persistent vomiting or diarrhea
9) Coughing or vomiting blood
10) Difficulty speaking
11) Unusual abdominal pain
12) Suicidal feelings, actions

WHEN SHOULD I CALL 911?

Before speeding to the ER yourself, you may benefit from calling 911 for immediate assistance. This call will help you assess the emergency and determine next, best steps. Call 911 if you suspect someone has a serious, life- or limb-threatening condition, or if the condition could significantly worsen while on the way to the ER, especially if traffic conditions could cause a delay or if moving the victim could cause more harm than good and require special skills or equipment—and if you're unsure what to do. When talking to a 911 operator, try to stay calm and speak clearly when explaining the emergency. Give your name and the phone number you're calling from and the exact address of the emergency. Answer the dispatcher's questions and follow their instructions. Don't hang up unless you are instructed to do so by the dispatcher, and don't leave the scene until help arrives. While waiting for the ambulance to arrive, it's helpful to gather all that you can, including the victim's list of medications, allergies, doctor's name and number, and insurance information. Obviously, if you are instructed to assist the victim with CPR or apply pressure to bleeding, don't leave that until the ambulance arrives.

WHEN IS IT MY TURN IN THE ER?

Emergency rooms do not work on patients on a first-come, first-serve basis. Thankfully, you don't have to take a number with a heart attack and get behind the guy with a minor injury! They work on a triage system. Triage comes from the French derivation, "to sort." Patients are categorized and seen according to the severity of their condition.

The triage nurse assesses your condition to determine its severity. Expect for your vital signs (heart rate, temperature and blood pressure, oxygen saturation called a pulse-ox) to be measured, along with other preliminary questions, which helps staff determine if you should be seen immediately or asked to wait, which should be a sort of relief. Many ERs have what's called a fast-track area to see and treat minor problems relatively quickly. This helps the ER address both the severe and less-severe patients rather efficiently. This goes for patients arriving in ambulances as well. Rest assured, you're not being overlooked, no matter how people arrive.

After triage, and once you are brought back to a room, a registration clerk will come in and get information such as date of birth, address, phone, name and number of doctor, and any insurance if you have it. You need to sign consent for treatment. In the room, you will probably see another nurse who works in the back and they, along with the treating doctors, will probably ask you the same questions. Don't be annoyed by the repetition. We know how information can be jumbled when in the midst of an emergency, so we are trained to be thorough.

WHAT'S TAKING SO LONG?

Instead of worrying about what's taking so long, be glad the medical staff is taking the necessary time to thoroughly review your condition and test results. Besides, if the condition is life- or limb-threatening, you will not be waiting. Here's what's happening behind the scenes.

After the doctor sees you, they order tests or do a procedure that could range widely, requiring time and attention. The reason you wait depends on several factors, such as how extensive the work-up is, how long the test results take to come back, whether another doctor or consultants is needed to see you, and how many other serious life- and limb-threatening conditions are being treated at the same time.

You would not want to be waiting during a heart attack or stroke for someone being treated for a broken arm or food poisoning. Emergency docs and nurses continue to triage care in the back and juggle all the conditions at once, which makes it stressful for them too.

Once your work-up is finished, the doctor will make a disposition, medical jargon for where you go next, which is basically one of two locations. You will either be discharged and go home—it can take some time to prepare the paperwork, instructions, and prescriptions, in addition to the verbal instructions and explanations the doctor and nurse will come to give you—or you will be admitted to the hospital for further treatment and monitoring. If you need admission but there are no beds available—which is a frequent issue for psychiatric patients but sometimes even for seriously ill patients waiting for an ICU bed—then you will stay in the ER because we can supply the levels of care of an ICU. And if it is overnight, this process is called boarding. Unfortunately, it sometimes can back-up the whole process for new patients coming in, but we continue to keep seeing everyone.

Nobody ever wants to go to the ER, and having a health emergency is extremely stressful. I hope this simplified explanation of what is going on behind the scenes can calm some of these fears and anxiety a bit. It's important to remember that if you do have a potentially life-threatening emergency, you will be taken care of first and that you are in good hands.

THE FATE OF US ALL

Another inevitable stress that we all must deal with, as Ben Franklin wrote in a letter to Jean-Baptiste Le Roy in 1789 "In this world nothing can be said to be certain except death and taxes." Death is one inevitable stress that we all have in common, no matter how hard we try to avoid it (especially since so many billionaires in the country seem to avoid paying their fair share of taxes, but that is a topic for another day).

As a child, losing my mom was one of my greatest fears. As an adult, as my mom's cancer took its toll, I knew her death was near, but I didn't want to face it. All too often, death knocks before we're ready. We never get to share our final words and feelings. Death has a way of stealing those moments because we weren't prepared, maybe too fearful of the awkward tension of planning for the inevitable. Death also has a way of putting life and what is really important into perspective. But even in the most horrible situations, sometimes you can find something humorous or something to celebrate.

When my mother passed away, it was the worst time of my life—something I'd worried about and dreaded since I was a little girl. It was my honor to take care of her during the last year of her life as she was dying of cancer. One of her final requests was to be buried with her cremated Shih Tzu Chu-Chee. Chu-Chee's remains had been saved inside a silk bag at my mom's house in Lake Placid.

On the day of the funeral, I wanted to sneak Chu-Chee into the casket next to my mom, so I asked her best friend from Lake Placid to bring her to the funeral. Although typical Jewish funerals don't have an open casket, we decided to allow a few of her very close friends and immediate family to see her one last time, since she had been living with me for her last year. While we were standing near the casket, my mom's friend Nita came in carrying a little wooden heart-shaped box.

"What's that and where's Chu-Chee?" I asked.

"This is it. This is what was in the urn," she said, as I opened up the box to find someone's stash of old marijuana!

"This obviously isn't Chu-Chee!" I said, bursting out laughing. "Her ashes were in a silk bag!"

"Well," my brother shot back, also cracking up, "I hope nobody was smoking Chu-Chee."

At this point, cannabis, including medical cannabis, was still illegal in Maryland. Frantically, my dad said, "We'd better put this away or we'll get arrested."

Needless to say, we did not bury the cannabis nor Chu-Chee with my mom. But we all couldn't help but have a good laugh despite our overwhelming grief, and she would have been laughing too!

My mom was the one who helped us all cope; while she was dying, she often told us she had no regrets, how much she loved us, and that she had a great life. I wrote her a letter that I was able to read to her the day before she died. Even as I read it, crying, she was comforting me, rubbing my arm and saying, "You don't have to say this, Leigh. I know how you feel, and you have shown me this our whole lives together."

After she died, when the rabbi came over to learn more about her, I read him the letter and he told me it was so beautiful that I should read it at her funeral, and I did. Here it is:

Dear Mom,

I know I don't have to tell you how I feel about you, but I want to tell you anyway, and I know that everything I am about to tell you, you would just say you already always knew. I thank God for being blessed with the most wonderful mother, and mother-daughter relationship, anyone could ask for. You are my best friend, my confidant, my mentor, my role model, and my idol. When I thought about it, there has not been a single day in my life that I did not talk with you at least once. Though most of my close friends and family know it has probably been many more times than once a day.

Even when I feel like I can't make a decision without you, you let me know that all you really did was support my choice . . . even when you disagreed. Your unconditional love and support have been my anchor all through my life. It has allowed me to achieve all that I have.

We never had those petty problems that other teenage girls had with their moms, to this day when I speak with mothers who have daughters and they tell me how difficult girls can be, I look at them in amazement, because I don't remember one teenage argument that I had with you. You were and still are the one person I could turn to with any problem or any question and know I would never be judged.

Your relationship with Popi Edi is truly a love match made in heaven, something I strive to emulate, together for over 35 years working and living together 24 hours a day. On the outside everyone thinks you called the shots, but we know that is just Ed's unassuming way. I know how much you love and respect him and how you never really make a move without getting his input and opinion.

Your relationship with Lary is also something I hope I have with my son when he grows up. Rarely have I seen a man who loves and cares for his mother as much as he does for you.

I remember our childhood filled with laughter, warmth, hugs and kisses. Even when I was mad at you for some silly thing, though not often, you would come into my room and kiss me until I erupted in giggles. I never could stay mad at you. Even when I said things I regretted later, you knew I didn't mean them; you were the one person who always understood my fears, my anger, my disappointment, and you could always help me work through them. In my 46 years of loving you, I got more than ten lifetimes worth of unconditional love and happiness. I hope I can be 1/1000 th the mother that you have been to me, and my son will be one very lucky little boy.

Speaking of you as grandmother, what child could ever have a better grandmother? Nana, for Max, the sun rises and sets in you. You are his whole world, and he's told me that you are the "best grandmother in the Milky Way." I know what he means to you; you once told me that you thought you could never love anyone as much as you loved Lary and me, but that was before you met him. There is so much of you I see in him too. Even at some of your sickest times this year, if he asked you to do something for him in school or elsewhere, you dragged yourself out of bed for him; you really are an amazing Nana.

Mom, the one thing this terrible cancer has given us is the gift of togetherness this past year. When you said to the doctor last week that you weren't ready for hospice care and "besides, who needs hospice, I have Leigh," it filled me with such pride. I want you to know that it has been my greatest pleasure and privilege in life to live with you these past 10 months and care for you.

I love you so much, Mom, even though I'm afraid that I can't make it without you and that has been the biggest fear my whole life...I know deep down that you have been such an outstanding mother and I know how well you've prepared me for life and motherhood . . . I don't want you to worry mom . . . I will be okay...and I will carry on your wonderful legacy...

Your Most Grateful, Loving Daughter,

Leigh

As hard as it was to say goodbye, my mom taught me that the sooner we prepare for this inevitable stress we will all have someday, the better. By formalizing our final wishes with respect to medical care, burials, wills, life insurance policies, as well as where to find these documents, we help lighten the load in future stressful situations for our loved ones, and what better gift to give them? In fact, during my mom's cancer treatments, I was afraid to bring all of this up—questions like where she wanted to be buried, here in Baltimore or back in Lake Placid? But she brought it up to me, to make it easier for me. All of this gave me one less thing to worry about. And again, she reminded me that she was okay with this all of this, that she'd had a wonderful life with my dad, my brother, and me, and her beloved grandson. Despite only a short 67 years on earth, she told me it felt like she'd had over 150 years worth of happiness.

There isn't a day that goes by that I don't miss and think about this remarkable woman. Despite my grief and feeling like the sun would never shine again, I was grateful for the time we had. In Judaism, after someone mentions the name of the deceased, they follow up with the words *zichronam livracha*,[96] which translate from Hebrew to English as: May their memory be a blessing. This type of grateful grieving will allow you to smile again while remembering your loved one, because their memory *is* a blessing.

However, one lesson that can be taken away from the Chu-Chee story is to make sure to leave explicit instructions on just what urn to look in!

Key Takeaways

- Life is full of inevitable stresses that we can't change; we need to understand how to manage them to help reduce our stress.
- You don't have to age gracefully; there is nothing wrong with spending time and/or money as well as taking pride in your appearance, because you are worth it.

- Understand your cancer and heart disease risks and modify your lifestyle; accordingly, women need to understand that our risk for developing heart disease is much higher than for breast cancer.
- Holidays can often be stressful with all the responsibilities, gifts, and meals falling on us. Do something different next year, such as taking a trip somewhere as a family and share an experience. That will last much longer than a physical gift or meal.
- Nobody expects to land in the ER, but sometimes we do; it's important to understand things can take time, and it's not first come, first serve, which is critical if you really are having a life-threatening problem. If this is the case you can rest assured that you will be taken first and that you are in good hands.
- We all eventually die, and as hard as it is, we can give ourselves and our loved ones peace of mind in the end by addressing important issues like how extensive our medical care should be in the end, as well as final burial wishes and where important documents are kept. This peace of mind will allow you to grieve with gratitude, so that their memory may be a blessing.

Chapter 9

Other Stress-Relieving Techniques

The only time we won't feel stress is when we're dead. In my life, whether I was waiting in the ER for an ambulance to deliver a patient or standing in the blocks waiting for the gun or whistle at the start of a track or swim race, I could feel the stress teeming through my body. It is the anticipation of not knowing what will come next that triggers our survival mechanism. As we discussed earlier in this book, this type of short-term stress can often be good; it gets you ready to jump into action, to save a life or win a race. But as you now know, over time, too much of a good thing wears down our bodies. Therefore, learning some simple techniques or seeking out regimens or treatment from experts can help you balance your life.

HUMAN TOUCH CAN WORK WONDERS

We humans are social animals; we need physical contact with others. We hug loved ones, shake hands with colleagues, get pats on the back for doing well. Human touch is incredibly important for our development and emotional well-being. Studies[1,2] on Romanian children in orphanages revealed that not being held as infants led to increased levels of the stress hormone cortisol, even until the age of 12 years old. This deprivation can lead to abnormal and lower levels of oxytocin, a feel-good hormone associated with emotional and social bonding, even after being adopted and three years of living with a family.[3]

We also know that skin-to-skin contact between mothers and their newborns shortly after birth is critical for both mother and child.[4] For babies, it helps regulate their breathing, heart rate, and feeding instinct. For moms, it helps boost milk supply. For both mom and baby, it releases that feel-good hormone oxytocin, that is so important in bonding.[5]

It isn't just children that can be soothed after a skinned knee from mom's embrace. Adults, too, can benefit from human touch. A large-scale review study done at the Netherland Institute for Neuroscience looked at 212 prior research studies and concluded that consensual touching can improve both your physical and mental well-being.[6] It was found to reduce pain as well as stress, anxiety, and depression—and increased frequency of touching had a greater impact. This makes sense because it is a part of social bonding.

We know interacting with people close to us is beneficial to our health and well-being. As we discussed before, social isolation and loneliness can put you at risk for cardiovascular disease and stroke, diabetes, anxiety, and depression.[7] This underscores the importance of reaching out to friends and family to talk about stressful issues in-person; know that their soothing caress is just as important as their sympathetic ear.

JOURNAL YOUR WAY OUT OF STRESS

Besides talking out your stresses, expressing yourself and your feelings by writing and keeping a journal can decrease stress and anxiety and help you manage traumas and anger. People who have experienced trauma talk about the cathartic effects of writing about it. It can make you more aware of feelings we sometimes suppress, and it can help you manage these emotions. It also stops the incessant dwelling on obsessive thoughts, which leads to anxiety. It is a form of journaling therapy.[8]

Other studies[9] found it can lead to fewer doctor's visits for stress-related problems, a decrease in work absenteeism, and improved mood with less depression and anxiety. Journaling was even found to improve physical parameters such as lung and liver function, decreased blood pressure, and improved immune function. In fact, another study[10] found that journaling, like art therapy, can reduce stress cortisol levels, which in turn reduce inflammatory cells; this was found to help wound healing in older adults.

We have already discussed how anger and resentment are harmful to your heart health, causing high blood pressure arrhythmias, and even dysfunction of blood vessels leading to clots[11]—not to mention the toll it takes on your mental health. Writing down those angry thoughts can help diffuse those feelings.

Flo, our adopted grandmother, who I mentioned earlier in the book, taught me the art of her "mad letters." Whenever she felt slighted or had an issue with a person or business, she would write a letter discussing the issue and her feelings and then send it via US mail. Even if she never heard back, the art of doing that helped her. It was probably not only writing down her feelings that was beneficial but sending it could have had benefits too.

A study published in *Nature Scientific Reports* found that participants who wrote down their angry thoughts after an insult and either threw them in the garbage or shredded them felt even better after disposing of the paper than the group that wrote down their thoughts and kept them in a file.[12] Perhaps after journaling those angry thoughts, you should rip out those pages, shred them, and dispose of them.

Of course, the converse is true. Feelings of gratitude for what we have and compassion toward others and ourselves can be beneficial for our physical and mental health.[13] Journaling those feelings is also very beneficial to your health; however, if you feel stressed about the idea of having to write out all your feelings, start out small. It does not have to be complicated long entries, just jotting down a few words from time to time about how you are feeling will get the ball rolling and be extremely helpful for your overall health!

TAP AWAY YOUR STRESS

I am not talking about tap dancing, although we know that dancing can be a great form of exercise, and that exercise is a great stress reliever. I am talking about Emotional Freedom Technique (EFT), a stress-relieving technique that involves tapping or pressing on points in the body that correspond to the same Chinese meridians points that are used in acupuncture. It got its start back in the 1970s and was refined and renamed EFT by Gary Craig in the 80s and 90s.[14]

The principle is similar to acupuncture in that it is supposed to create energy balance that can reduce your stress and help with anxiety, as well as pain. The twelve meridians are believed to stimulate sensory nerves and signal the brain to cause these clinical changes.[15] There are websites that can better describe the technique and show you exactly what to do and where to tap.[16]

Generally, there are several steps, starting with determining what is making you anxious and upset. You need to rank how intense these feeling are on a scale from 1 to 10 so that you can monitor your progress. You must also create a couple of phrases identifying the problem but also forgiving and accepting yourself and your feelings, such as, "Even though I am stressed about [fill in the blank], I still acknowledge and accept how I am feeling." You then begin tapping seven times on each area, starting with the pinkie side of your hands, while repeating the phrase; you then move on to your eyebrows, the sides of your eyes, under your eyes, under your nose, your chin, on your collar bone, and under your arms, finishing on top of your head. You do this, repeating your phrase and maintaining the focus on your issue. At the end of the sequence, you reassess how you are feeling.

While I know some doctors think this is pseudoscience, there are clinical trials that have shown benefits. A recent randomized controlled trial[17] done during COVID-19, looking at nurses and their stress and anxiety while working during the pandemic, found the group that did online EFT had reduced stress anxiety and lower burnout levels than the control group, who did not practice this technique.

Another study done on nursing students[18] also found it was an effective stress-reduction tool that helped reduce anxiety. One review study found it was effective at decreasing depressive symptoms;[19] another found it could improve self-esteem.[20] Another one looked at the mechanism of action by evaluating psychological factors and physiologic parameters to measure the benefits for stress reduction.[21]

After a four-day workshop done in different locations, participants had both physiological factors such as resting pain level, heart rate, blood pressure, and cortisol levels. They also had psychological testing done to assess anxiety, depression, even perceived happiness. What the researchers found was improvements in resting heart rate, a decrease in blood pressure, positive trends in heart rate variability (which is a measure of cardiovascular fitness), cortisol levels decreased by 37 percent. At just one workshop 40 percent of participants reported a decrease in anxiety, a 35 percent reported a decrease in depression, 57 percent reported decreased pain, and over one-third reported feeling happier. This technique really has no downside or potential complications, so give it a try when you are feeling stressed!

HOW ABOUT THOSE MERIDIANS FOR ACUPUNCTURE?

Acupuncture has been a part of Chinese medicine for over 3,000 years.[22] While modern Western medicine is slowly starting to embrace it, we are still trying to understand the physiologic mechanisms of how it works. There are studies[23] that show acupuncture can cause increased levels in our brain and bloodstream of our natural pain-reducing compounds called endorphins and enkephalins.

Additionally, it can boost levels in the brain of the neurotransmitters that regulate anxiety, such as serotonin and dopamine. This is why it is useful in the treatment of painful conditions like migraines, fibromyalgia, and arthritis as well as anxiety and depression. There is also a synergy of the therapeutic effects of acupuncture with our endocannabinoid system that regulate stress as well.[24]

A large review study looking at acupuncture use for anxiety in humans and animals found that despite the varied methodology of the different clinical trials, there still was evidence that it was effective at reducing stress and anxiety. [25] In fact, the study noted that it was comparable to cognitive behavioral therapy (CBT), which is the standard psychological type of talk therapy aimed at teaching coping skills to change behaviors and thoughts. Another acupuncture study done in rats looked at anxiety related to nicotine withdrawal.[26] Researchers found it could change the levels of a hormone, corticotrophin-releasing factor (CRF) in the amygdala, the part of the brain that processes fear and our fight-or-flight response. CRF regulates cortisol levels in the body and by reducing the levels of the stress hormone cortisol, it was found to attenuate the anxiety response seen during nicotine withdrawal.

When looking at people with post-traumatic stress disorder (PTSD), it was also found to be more beneficial than doing nothing, and as beneficial as CBT with the effects lasting at their three-month follow-up.[27] Another study done on healthcare providers using auricular (ear) acupuncture at relaxation points found it had anti-anxiety effects, along with decreased heart rate and blood pressure when compared to the placebo group, which had sham needles placed in fake pressure points in the ear.[28] Acupuncture for anxiety had fewer side effects than medications used to treat anxiety.[29] So the next time you are feeling stressed, find a licensed acupuncturist and try being a pincushion, because it really doesn't even hurt!

TURN YOURSELF INWARD

Mindfulness and meditation have always been a part of Eastern medicine, and like acupuncture, Western medicine is starting to better understand and take notice. Mindfulness and meditation are complex neurophysiological processes that involves many different areas of the brain affecting our thoughts and cognition and our sensory perception. It affects our autonomic nervous system and the areas in the brain controlling our sympathetic nervous system; they are turned down along with our flight-or-fight response[30] while activating our para-sympathetic nervous system, which functions during times of rest and relaxation, sometimes called the rest and digest response.[31] It can lower our heart rate and blood pressure,[32] as well as cortisol levels.[33] Meditation has also been found to help with chronic pain and the depressive symptoms related to it.[34]

A study done on college students experiencing stress with perfectionism leading to anxiety and depression found improvement after two semesters of Transcendental Meditation (TM).[35] This is another indication that being a perfectionist is a stressful burden. Another interesting study done in college students found that meditation can not only lower stress levels, but it also enhanced forgiveness,[36] something we all need to practice more. Forgiveness, as we discussed prior in the book, also has stress-relieving benefits.

A review study that looked at over thirty-six randomized controlled trials, the gold standard for research, examined different meditative practices and their effect on anxiety. Researchers found meditation to be a useful and effective tool in reducing the symptoms of anxiety.[37]

Another review study, looking at more than 600 different studies on transcendental meditation, found it was more effective than many other types of alternative treatments, such as exercise, especially in patients with high anxiety levels, such as those with chronic anxiety disorder, veterans with PTSD, and prison inmates.[38] Their findings showed reduction of symptoms within the first two weeks and sustained effects for three years. By practicing mindfulness and meditating, we can improve both our physical and mental health.

Besides reducing stress, it can improve our cognition and attention, create greater compassion and forgiveness, and even improve sleep.[39] Therefore, the next time you feel stressed, take a beat, slow down a bit, and turn your focus inward.

FOLLOW YOUR PASSION

It isn't a surprise that work-related stress can be a tough challenge to deal with, and we have discussed the health ramifications earlier in the book. According to the American Psychological Association,[40] it is the second most common stress people report, with over 60 percent saying it is one of their biggest stresses. An eight-decade study done at the University of California, Riverside[41] found that people who are passionate about their work were more productive and good at their jobs; in fact, they lived longer than those who were laid back. Part of it is that their work makes them happy, and studies find that that leads to less stress and a longer life.[42] And the converse is true too. A study found women in lower-level routine jobs had lower life expectancy and more unhappiness and stress.[43]

It doesn't have to be passion just about your work. Volunteering for causes you are passionate about may have the same effects. Research out of the University of Michigan[44] found that selfless volunteering can lengthen your life. It fills your life with purposeful meaning. But the caveat is that you need to do it for the right reasons; it can't be for self-serving reasons, but for true selfless passion for your cause with the idea of helping other—true altruism.

DON'T BE AFRAID TO SUCK AT SOMETHING NEW

It's human nature to have fears; in fact, fear is part of our fight-or-flight response, and it is a defense mechanism needed for survival.[45] But just like the stress response that becomes dangerous when chronic, so does fear. Constant irrational fear and the ensuing anxiety can become a pathological phobia. Despite some research stating that most phobias begin in childhood and have a genetic familial base, that only partly explains them, and often the individual's person experience is a more reliable predictor.[46] This is good news because it means we can often take control of our fears! Frequently, the absolute best way to ease the fear is to face it head-on.

I remember when my son was just three years old, and he wanted to join the cannonball contest at our community pool with the older kids. He could not swim well yet and he was wearing swim floaties on each arm. His father tried to discourage him because he was slightly frightened jumping off the diving board for the first time even though they were going to allow me to be in the water to catch him.

I told him to give it try, that he knew he could float in the deep end with his floaties and me in the pool nearby. (I always recommend to moms: Never use a flotation device in place of careful supervision.) He had done that before even though it was not off the diving board. Well, he did it, made it to the side without me even catching him, and I remember how proud he felt when he won a ribbon in his age class, since he was the only toddler to enter!

He was so excited when he told me, "Mom, at first I was afraid like Dad, but then I did it like you, a brave Vinocur, and now I am not afraid anymore to try things!"

Then he spent the whole afternoon jumping off the diving board, which meant I was in the water all day that day! Now, don't get me wrong. As I stated earlier in the book, as an ER doctor, I am trained to consider the worst-case scenarios. Therefore, I do not recommend that you become a fearless risk-taker trying dangerous feats. The point is that when we tell ourselves scary stories that prevent us from acting, we sometimes realize the fears, and related stress, were blown out of proportion. If and when the next situation arises where fears dominate, we can find strength in our ability to face it because we've done it before. Facing fears can harness the stress for success!

That is why I stated that you should try something new, a challenge even if you are not sure it is something you can do. Trying new things that are uncomfortable (not dangerous) and out of your wheelhouse even if you think you will stink/suck at it, once completed with good or bad results, still helps you develop self-esteem. And that is good for you. Studies find there is a positive psychology behind overcoming new challenges.[47]

Whenever we anticipate doing something new, we can feel trepidation or apprehension because it's unfamiliar and we don't want to fail, or even look like a failure. But those fears are often the opposite of what people think. Instead, people will label you as courageous.

As far as my career, I have always used my medical degree to challenge myself and try different complementary adjunct career paths. Besides practicing emergency medicine and urgent care, running fifteen clinics in the mid-Atlantic, I have an adjunct medical broadcasting career. I have worked as a chief medical officer overseeing the science department and research in both the biomedical device industry and the nutraceutical industry.

Most recently, as I am writing this, I am opening a new men's health clinic, going back to my urology roots. Additionally, a few years ago I got my master's degree in medical cannabis science and therapeutics and started a small cannabis medical practice and consulting firm that I still have. Each time embarking on a new opportunity, I was not sure if I would succeed but feel accomplished just by trying something new. I love it, because as I said before, I consider myself a lifelong learner and I do love learning new things! Even just writing this book was a scary endeavor; I wasn't sure how it would turn out and if it would suck! But I had to do it, even just to prove to myself that I was resilient and up to the challenge. With each new challenge, it became a little easier to do the next. So I want to encourage you to be brave enough to suck at something new. It will increase your self-confidence and break down those fears in the future.

I am not advocating completely ditching a career that you spent years training for, like medicine or law, to open a mushroom farm, unless, of course, you are truly miserable. Even in that event, I always started slowly, maintaining my day job while learning that new skill. I am sure there are skills you've learned along your career path that can serve you in other areas. Finding something new you enjoy can open avenues to consider a completely new career path. For example, if mushroom farming is it, explore this as a new hobby and star out small, before you bet the whole farm on it, so to speak!

NEW HOBBIES

This gives you lots of options to suck at something new while experiencing something you've always wanted to do. And it doesn't have to be for a new career path; it can be anything that challenges you to try something new and out of your typical comfort range. Some examples:

- Learn a new language, join a language club to practice with, or take that trip to France or Italy.
- Find a new book club or take an evening literature class at a local college.
- Take sports lessons; try golf, snowboarding, or pickle ball, and join a league.

We already discussed the stress-reducing benefits of charitable work; I have friends that, through their passionate work with charity, actually found new careers that give them a more meaningful and purposeful life, as well as a surefire way harness their stress. As we have stated before, when focusing on compassionate ways to serve others, often the fear of trying something new disappears.

TRY PUBLIC SPEAKING

Public speaking is widely known to be one of our greatest fears and sources of stress and social anxiety,[48] but it also proves a useful tool in anything you choose to do with your life. At one point or another, whether it is a work presentation, standing up at a school board meeting, or a speaking at a charity committee that you serve on, someone may ask you to give a talk. This is one of the best ways to get you a little out of your comfort zone and try some new things.

Studies find that over 25 percent of people say public speaking is one of their top fears.[49] For many, the mere thought of being under the spotlight, in front of people who are examining every word, is enough freak them out. Of course, it's natural that it is uncomfortable at first, but once you do it, you gain confidence,[50] and by overcoming and facing that fear, you will always come out on top, regardless of what you thought the outcome was. The reality is that you always perform better than you think, because we are our worst critics. Most audiences appreciate us as human beings and don't look to judge or condemn us, as we naturally fear they are doing.

While there are many things you can learn to become a better speaker, here are a few guidelines to relieve the stress of being on stage:

- Be yourself, and speak conversationally; if you stumble a bit, that is natural and human—nobody wants to listen to a robot.
- Be professional; depending on your audience, you may want to avoid casual or work-specific jargon. Avoid slang and profanity as well.
- Be prepared; this is the best way to relieve the stress associated with public speaking. That means practice, but nobody cares if you bring a few note cards with your key points outlined as long as you try not to read from them.
- Be clear and enunciate; don't rush your speaking pattern.
- Be interesting; start off with an attention-grabbing story, joke, or factoid.

If you are still worried, consider taking a public speaking class at a local college or even joining an organization like Toastmasters, which also offers education programs.[51] Conquering a fear of public speaking is one of the best ways to enhance self-confidence and boost self-esteem, and you will gain a huge sense of accomplishment.

Something magical happens when you're in front of an audience who wants to hear from you. You become the expert, with power to influence. Still, it can be a frightening thought for anyone, and there is always that little voice in your heading worrying about the worst possible outcome. But that's why getting involved in networking groups and practicing can help you face the fear of public speaking and walk away better for it. This applies to other fears, stresses, and anxieties as well. The more often we step out of our comfort zone, the more comfortable we become with the process. Trying new things can be exciting.

FIND YOUR SPIRITUAL CENTER

When my mother was in her final days, I was overcome with fears of the unknown. My greatest fear in my life was losing her. How would I continue without my greatest confidant, my strongest supporter and best friend? I wondered about life after her death, and what my life was all about. I have a Jewish background, and while not very religious, I've always been very spiritual, as was my mom. However, when I was faced with this kind of anxiety, I did return to more traditional religious roots to help me find my spiritual center.

I found a Tehillim prayer group where women come together and pray for those sick in the community through the Book of Psalms—aka Tehillim. I started going weekly and met so many wonderful, supportive women all going through different things and all with amazing stories. We, as a group, prayed for healing of the sick among other things, while reading the Book of Psalms written by King David.[52] One day, I'd like to write about the experience, but for now I'll just say it was good for the soul. So good, in fact, to this day I keep going to the group when I can even after my mom died.

There are some studies that talk about how it is scientifically impossible to accurately measure the power of prayer and if it shows merit,[53] but as physician, I have seen improvements and recoveries in patients that cannot be explained medically. A case report of a sixteen-year-old with a chronic gastrointestinal problem required tube feeding since birth that resolved completely after proximal prayer during a church service.[54]

Another study, published in the prestigious *British Medical Journal (BMJ)* from 2001, looked at over 3,000 patients, randomizing them, which is considered the most valued type of medical trial, to two groups, a prayer group or no prayer group. The researchers found that those in the prayer group had shorter hospital stays with less blood infections and lower mortality after trauma.[55]

Some scientists think prayer is akin to meditation, which has healing benefits, but whether you believe it or not, as the researchers pointed out, it has no side effects, so there really is no downside to trying it. When my mom was dying, even though I was going to a Jewish prayer group, my best friend and her mother had nuns praying for my mom; my feeling was that the more prayers, the better, no matter who was praying. Alas, you know that she died anyway; but that does not dampen my spirituality, which I feel has helped me cope with many different stresses and obstacles in life.

WHEN MORE THAN STRESS AND PROFESSIONAL HELP IS NEEDED

When it goes beyond stress and becomes a serious condition of anxiety and/or depression, there is no shame in that diagnosis. In fact, according to the CDC, over 20 percent, that is one in five Americans, experience mental illness,[56] with almost one-quarter of women in the US suffering from mental illness.[57] When that is your diagnosis, then no amount of baking, decorating, clearing out clutter, taking a hot bath, getting high on nature, or my stress-reducing tips will help.

This book is not intended to be a treatment guide for psychiatric illness as I am not a psychiatrist. However, as an emergency physician, I have spent much of my 30 years in practice caring for patients during experiencing psychiatric emergencies. Unfortunately, due to a lack of an adequate number of psychiatric beds in hospitals across the country, these poor patients in crisis often have to be kept in the ER, sometime for days and weeks while waiting for placement. This is both dangerous for the psychiatric patient and the ER, as it cripples flow for new patients coming in.[58] So, I have taken care of my fair share of these patients.

The unfortunate truth is that stress leading to anxiety and depression can be dangerous and should not be taken lightly. Serious depression can lead us to think we are hopeless, that life is not worth living and that our loved ones would be better off without us. Sadly, women attempt suicide two to four times more often than men.[59] But it doesn't have to go there. We have options, and while previously in the book I discussed when you should seek professional help, I want to end this chapter by addressing some of these options and possible interventions so that you can discuss them with your health care provider. While it is not an exhaustive, in-depth list, it is a starting point. I always believe that knowledge is power; the more you know, the better off you are.

COGNITIVE BEHAVIORAL THERAPY

As a physician, as with any medical intervention, I always recommend starting with the most conservative, least-invasive procedures and treatments. In physical ailments, my feeling is that surgery should be the last resort; the same goes for psychiatric treatment. Therefore, one of the first steps and very effective therapeutic options to consider is cognitive behavioral therapy (CBT), a form of talk psychotherapy aimed at behavioral modification.

CBT was pioneered in the 1960's by Dr. Aaron Beck.[60, 61] He noticed that many of his depressed patients expressed that they had distorted cognitive thoughts running through their minds that were not being addressed with the traditional psychoanalysis, which tends to blame everything on your childhood! Since that time, studies numbering over 2,000 have found that CBT is an effective therapy[62] to help people manage the maladaptive thoughts they have that leads to their behaviors.

In fact, we know it is more often than not our interpretation of a situation that influences our emotional and psychological state and leads to our behaviors. By discussing and identifying these often-irrational thoughts and beliefs about yourself, hopefully you can cognitively change your outlook and thus your behavior, which will in turn help you deal with your anxiety and depression. A good CBT therapist will give you tools to use when that voice in your head is perpetuating those thoughts and anxieties.

PHARMACOTHERAPY WITH ANTIDEPRESSANTS

Sometimes CBT alone is not enough. So the next least-invasive thing to consider might be medication. Today we know that there is a neurochemical basis for depression and anxiety. Some people have chemical imbalances in the brain that benefit from medications.

The pharmacotherapeutic basis of depression and anxiety is related to a depletion and lower levels of important brain neurotransmitters/neurochemicals such as serotonin, norepinephrine, and dopamine.[63] That is why there are antidepressant and anti-anxiety medications that many patients are prescribed for both anxiety and depression, that inhibit the depletion or re-uptake of these neurochemicals, increasing their level in the brain. Examples of some common medications used for both anxiety and depression are fluoxetine, brand name Prozac, and sertraline, brand name Zoloft; they are selective serotonin reuptake inhibitors (SSRIs). Another is duloxetine, brand name Cymbalta; it is a selective serotonin and norepinephrine reuptake inhibitor (SNRI).

There are studies that find using pharmacotherapy in combination with CBT can be beneficial.[64] We still need to learn resilience when we feel beaten down, and coping skills when our minds are racing, and have our tool bag full of all available resources. That's why I'm a believer in simultaneous medication and talk therapy like CBT.

MEDICAL CANNABIS THERAPEUTICS

As I stated, part of my try-something-new recommendation, several years ago I went back to school and got one of the first master's degrees in the country in medical cannabis science and therapeutics. As I described earlier in the book, we have our own internal neuromodulating physiological system called the endocannabinoid system (ECS). We make our own cannabinoid molecules that essentially affect and regulate almost every biologic function in our body.

One internal cannabinoid or endocannabinoid that our body synthesizes during times of stress is called anandamide;[65] it calms our nervous system down and is called our "bliss molecule." The other is called arachidonoylglycerol (2-AG).[66] Human studies have found that dysfunction in the ECS can affect our mood and contribute to anxiety and depression. They also interact with the receptors in the brain that regulate the same neurotransmitters as serotonin and norepinephrine.[67] This is why many people turn to cannabis to treat their anxiety and depression.

Plant cannabinoids such as THC and CBD can also interact with the key brain neurochemical receptors that play a role in anxiety and depression, such as serotonin; however, it can be dose-dependent for THC products. Low doses can have anti-anxiety and antidepressant effects, while high doses can actually trigger anxiety and depression.[68] An older study from the 1980s found that CBD can have anti-anxiety properties in both low and high doses and can mitigate anxiety produced from THC as well as its intoxicating effects.[69] That is why it is very important to talk with a physician or mental health professional who is educated in medical cannabis if you are having symptoms of anxiety and depression. You should not self-medicate with cannabis but use it under a clinician's supervision! But you should also know because it is still federally illegal and only certain states have enacted medical cannabis laws depending on where you live in the US, getting this treatment will depend on your access to medical cannabis therapeutics and having knowledgeable health care providers.

PSYCHEDELIC-ASSISTED THERAPY

The next potential newer therapy is the use of the psychedelic drug ketamine. Often it is administered intravenously and is reserved for treatment-resistant depression. Ketamine is an anesthetic from the 1960s that is still sometimes used in the emergency department for short procedures like relocating a patient's dislocated shoulder. This is because it has dissociative effects, causing amnesia so that the patient will not recall the procedure. The IV form, which is given in sub-anesthetic doses, has not been approved by the FDA for this type of psychiatric treatment.[70] There is one form, a nasal spray, that has been FDA-approved for treatment-resistant depression.[71]

The way ketamine works is different than other antidepressants; it triggers a chemical called glutamate that allows the brain to make new nerve connections to help patients develop more positive behaviors and attitudes.[72] While it is a relatively newer treatment for serious depression, several studies show ketamine-assisted therapy can quickly lower stress and depression while regenerating areas of the brain causing the symptoms.[73,74, 75] If it works, patients find that it does so much faster than traditional antidepressants. While some patients call this a miracle drug, I have seen patients for whom it has not worked at all.

We must remember that no medicine is 100 percent safe. All medications, whether synthetic from pharmaceutical companies or natural like cannabis, do have a risk-benefit ratio. And they cannot solve all our problems; therefore, we must be realistic about our risk and reward ratio.

TRANSCRANIAL MAGNETIC STIMULATION (TMS)

The next level of treatment is Transcranial Magnetic Stimulation (TMS), a procedure that uses a magnetic field to stimulate nerve cells in the brain. It was FDA-approved in 2008 to treat very difficult cases of depression and obsessive-compulsive disorder (OCD), which is a specialized, severe form of anxiety disorder. While the mechanism of how TMS works is still not fully understood, there are postulated theories that the magnetic field creates an electrical current causing a change in the metabolic activity in the brain.[76]

TMS is a noninvasive procedure that must be performed in a physician's office. It involves delivering repetitive magnetic pulses to the exterior of the scalp. There are no negative side effects, and it does not require sedation or anesthesia. There may be some scalp tingling and twitching of facial muscle and nerves.

For OCD, which can be a very hard-to-treat and disabling condition, causing intrusive thoughts and behaviors like constant hand washing, studies have shown that up to 45 to 55 percent of patients had reduced symptoms one month after treatment.[77,78]

CRANIAL ELECTROTHERAPY STIMULATION (CES)

Another type of electrotherapy is Cranial Electrotherapy Stimulation (CES). It is a painless, effective adjunctive treatment for insomnia, anxiety, depression, and PTSD.[79,80,81] Using a low-intensity electrical current delivered from electrodes attached, typically to the earlobes or temples, the treatment aims to modulate—or balance—the central and peripheral nervous system.

The resulting effects stimulate the brain to produce and maintain serotonin levels, as well as other neurochemicals required for healthy mood and sleep, while also entraining a calm brainwave state and modulating the fight-or-flight sympathetic nervous system. Perhaps the best part is that you can literally use a device at home; however, the FDA-cleared class II device has been shown to be effective, but it does require a physician's prescription.

ELECTROCONVULSIVE THERAPY (ECT)

Lastly, the most invasive electrotherapy is one of oldest methods used in psychiatry. First introduced in Rome in 1937,[82] electroconvulsive therapy (ECT) passes an electrocurrent through the head, intentionally causing a brief seizure. It has been portrayed in movies, and while it is not as bad as Hollywood depicts, it is an invasive procedure. It is safer today, using lower current requiring general anesthesia, which has its own inherent risks.

Since there are other similar therapies like TMS and CES, ECT has been falling out of favor. It is believed to work by increasing key neurotransmitters like serotonin in the brain and creating new connections between nerve cells.[83] But it is often considered a last-resort therapy for those intractable, difficult-to-treat cases of severe depression, and even psychotic conditions such as schizophrenia.[84]

Key Takeaways

- The human touch can do wonders for stress, so reach out to family and friends when you need a hug.
- Expressing your feelings by writing them down in a journal is a cathartic way to manage your stress.
- Tapping is an easy technique you can learn to help manage stress; it utilizes the acupuncture meridians.
- Also consider seeing a licensed acupuncturist; studies and 3,000 years of Eastern medicine find that it can help you manage stress.
- Practicing mindfulness and meditation and turning your thoughts inward is also great stress reliever.
- Following your passion, whether in a career or a charity you volunteer for, can center you; in essence, concentrating on the others you are helping helps you and relieves stress.

- Don't be afraid to try to learn something new; it can be a hobby or sport or even a class on something like public speaking. While everyone worries about failure, pushing through those fears will do wonders for building your self-confidence and self-esteem.
- Finding your spiritual center can help with stress and anxiety. Studies have found the power of prayer can be a form of meditation.
- If all your stresses become too much, *do not* be ashamed to ask for professional help. It is critical to discuss your options with an expert, and as with any medical condition, always start with the least invasive therapeutic options first.

Chapter 10

Topping It Off

Driving down the highway in the dark, I was exhausted. I was returning home from a 15-minute meeting in New Jersey. I had been asked to attend by our sales rep to explain the benefits my company's high-quality saw palmetto extract has on the prostate gland to a urologist. It was an almost four-hour drive each way, and I had already been driving nearly eight hours that day— no wonder I was feeling exhausted. But wanting to get more done that day, I juggled phone calls on the way back, including one from the sales rep. Sounding grateful, he assured me it had been well-worth everyone's time that I'd made the drive. I secretly questioned this.

As the drive droned on, I started wondering how much longer it would be until my exit came up. I had made the drive from my home in Maryland to New Jersey many times, so I started to look out for anything familiar. I kept driving and driving. Another 20 minutes went by, and I had to admit I was lost!

That's it, I thought. *I have Alzheimer's and soon I'll be drooling in the corner and won't be able to remember my son's name!*

I called Tony, who was expecting me home 30 minutes earlier. "I don't know where I'm at!" He said he'd tracked my phone and couldn't figure out why I went past the exit and started heading toward the I-70, and asked, "What have you been doing?"

"Well, I was on the phone," I said, admittedly shook up, thinking I was losing my marbles.

"Leigh," he replied, "you're just not paying attention. You need to turn around and focus on your driving."

Easier said than done. First, I can't see well at night since I have mono-vision contacts, which my optometrist said makes my far vision not optimal.

Secondly, I had a million things going on in my head. I realized I must have been thinking I was heading west on the beltway instead of east from I-95.

In the end, I made it home safe—but I still believed I might be one step closer to dementia. Looking back, I was scared. I was tired. I felt like I had wasted a lot of time that day. I just wanted to be in my bathtub, soaking away the stresses of the day.

This really gave credence to the adage, "Live in the moment and be present." Well, that sounds wonderful, but the truth is, sometimes we feel like we're trapped in the moment. Despite our best efforts, we feel like it's all we can do just to survive the moment. We put so much pressure on ourselves, we expect so much that we don't give ourselves a break—especially when we need it the most. We can get tunnel vision when we need broad vision. Our feelings can get in the way when they don't need to. We can stress ourselves out when there's really no need to be stressed.

The fact is the urologist *did* listen to me, the sales rep *was* pleased I made the journey, I *did* make good use of my time on the road, and I wasn't really needed at home that day. I needed to let go of my own expectations, give myself a little latitude, as well as be more present, especially when driving! Instead of trying to cram all the other things on my list into that eight-hour drive, I should have just turned on my Bluetooth Spotify to listen to music that I loved and chilled out during that drive.

We all feel like our daily stresses can makes us freaking crazy. But we must keep it all in perspective so it doesn't keep us from what matters to us. Often, we are the ones putting the added pressure on ourselves, becoming our own worst enemy. We need to learn how to say no to the things that don't really matter to us and our loved ones that we sometimes get roped into. That's why I want to leave you with the following words of advice, which I've learned through my various career reinventions, workplace bullying, motherhood madness, and from my beloved and wise mom:

Believe in yourself. Sounds cliché, but it is true. Regardless of what the world and these crazy times throw at us, there is nobody better at being you than you.

You have to think you can; otherwise you will live a self-fulfilling prophecy and surely disappoint yourself. Remember the story about when I entered college, and my interview counselor told me she was surprised my SAT scores were not that high considering I had all As and ranked in the top five of my class in high school? She told me that I would do well at Michigan but that I shouldn't pick a career in medicine because of my standardized testing scores. But I believed that I could do anything I wanted. And I did.

I believed I could learn just about anything in my field and become an expert. Working in the emergency department helped strengthen this belief because we had to take care of every kind of medical problem that walked in that door, and at a moment's notice. The same goes for being a medical expert reporting in the media. I knew I could answer any question thrown to me in an interview. While new experiences help build the belief in yourself, the belief must come first. If I didn't believe I could be a doctor, I never would have tried, let alone made it. Believing in yourself may sound trivial, but it is not; it is critical to building your self-esteem and accomplishing the goals you set for yourself.

Learn to advocate for yourself. You must become your own best advocate. Men do it all the time. For some reason, women feel like it would be bragging or tooting their own horns. I'm not suggesting becoming a narcissist who only thinks of themselves. I'm talking about being aware of opportunities, creating your own, and communicating your talents and assets with confidence. In fact, an article written in *Harvard Business Review*[1] reported prior research that found women will only apply for jobs when they are 100 percent qualified, whereas men will apply for jobs if they feel they are at least 60 percent qualified. Men don't worry about over-promising and under-delivering. This says a lot about the confidence men have in themselves, and how women really sell themselves short, because we know no one is ever 100 percent qualified!

I remember when my Medical College Admission Test (MCAT) scores came back, and I was not even granted an interview for my alma mater University of Michigan. While memories of what that interview counselor told me about not getting into medicine four years earlier could have easily kept me stuck in my tracks, I did not let them. I marched into the admissions office without a scheduled interview and didn't leave until I had what I wanted. I told them, "I'm a top Michigan graduate with all As, my dad went to medical school here, and just because I don't do well with standardized tests like the MCAT, it shouldn't prevent me from at least the courtesy of an interview, before they say no." Well, they did give me an interview, and I was then put on their waitlist. However, by then I had accepted admission to another medical school… their loss!

Don't be afraid to take risks. Another cliché that rings true is, "You have to put yourself out there," but not on a limb or plank. I'm talking about taking calculated risks that have minimal if any downsides. Why not go for it? If we don't, we'll never know, because nobody else is going to take the initiative for us.

Of course, taking risks is easier if you believe in, and can advocate for, yourself. And there's always something to be learned if you do take the risk. If successful, you'll end up growing in confidence as a result. That new job opportunity or new responsibility at work may not be there if you wait until you feel you meet 100 percent of the criteria. Don't let the fear of taking it on, even with the possibility of overpromising and underdelivering, stop you.

Men don't seem to let these fears prevent them from going for it. They would never let an opportunity for advancement go by, worrying about if they can deliver. Most jump and say yes and then figure out the how later, learning on the fly. Why shouldn't we do this too?

Every time I've made a career move, from medicine to broadcast to the medical cannabis or nutraceutical/biotech industries—I've even been a crime scene investigator, because I love forensic medicine—I made the change, but I did not have previous experience in any of these areas. You might have to read that sentence again, but it's true. I decided that I wanted to try something new and expand my knowledge and my world, so I went for it and let the chips fall into place. I had to learn on the fly and bounce back from failures and mistakes. If you don't take risks, you never have the chance at the rewards.

Learn to accept (even welcome) rejection and failure. For every opportunity I've had, I've had twice as many rejections and failures. I've had many doors slammed in my face. Of course, it was disappointing, but with persistence, perseverance, and sometimes with a little luck, a door will finally open.

I learned along the way that these failures and disappointments taught me about resilience, one of the most powerful attributes I developed. I always say that breaking into medical broadcasting was harder than getting into medical school. I pounded the pavement, kept calling news directors for years. Finally, I broke through in Baltimore's WBAL TV. My persistence of calling their new news director, and leaving my number every week, paid off. After a CSX train derailment in Baltimore, he called me at the last minute to comment on the repercussions of a toxic spill after the derailment.

He was impressed that I could go on air and discuss a toxic spill's potential health implications with only three minutes' notice. I told him it was just like in the ER, I have to be ready to take care of any critical patients that come through the doors; late-breaking medical news was the same. He told me to come in the next the morning and hired me right then as a morning medical news reporter/contributor.

You don't need to fear failure and rejection. But you do need to learn from them. You can't take it personally, and you have to shut out the voice that says, *You are not good enough.* Instead, turn this thought on its head by thinking, *This opportunity was not good for me. They did not see my capabilities, so I'm going to move on.*

I remember one of my best, most expensive failures: an informatics company I helped build with another physician friend, my partner Tony, and a few software developers. We all hoped to help lower healthcare costs while practicing evidence-based medicine. It was a clinical decision support tool that could be applied to any electronic medical record (EMR) system. It could notify doctors with real-time comparative costs for best practices in clinical action. For example, it would let you see comparative pricing on all the different effective recommended medications for a specific type of illness.

We had pilot programs going in two significant healthcare networks and I busted my butt, investing time, sweat equity, and over $35,000 to bring it to market. But a huge EMR company got ahold of our proprietary software, stole it, and published a white paper saying how they could integrate it into their platform. Our dreams soon faded, and the start-up business came to a screeching halt.

Despite the company going under, it was a great learning experience that I would not change. I take pride in knowing we built something that the biggest EMR company in the US was actually threatened by! We had failed, but I did as my grandmother used to sing to me—from a 1930s Fred Astaire movie— "You just pick yourself up and dust yourself off and start all over again!"

If there's one thing, I hope you remember from reading this book, it is to give yourself a break. Be kind to yourself; you deserve some grace and understanding. You are capable of so much more than you give yourself credit for. Life is full of stressful moments. But just like my exit when driving back from New Jersey, they will pass by too! You are still the best person in the world to be you. And the world needs you, whether or not they see you sweat.

Notes

INTRODUCTION

1. Bazyar J et al. Triage Systems in Mass Casualty Incidents and Disasters: A Review Study with A Worldwide Approach. *Open Access Maced J Med Sci.* 2019; 7(3):482–494.

2. Vinocur L. Prioritizing mental health shouldn't be risky for physicians, *MedpageToday.* July 22, 2020. https://www.medpagetoday.com/publichealthpolicy/generalprofessionalissues/87685. Accessed June 18, 2024.

3. Infurna F et al. Historical change in midlife health, well-being, and despair: Cross-cultural and socioeconomic comparisons. *Am Psychol.* 2021; 76(6):8 70-887.

4. Yim J. Therapeutic Benefits of Laughter in Mental Health: A Theoretical Review. *Tohoku J Exp Med.* 2016 Jul;239(3):243–249.

5. Güler O, et. al. Positive Psychological Impacts of Cooking During the COVID-19 Lockdown Period: A Qualitative Study. *Front Psychol.* 2021 Mar 18;12:635957. doi: 10.3389/fpsyg.2021.635957. PMID: 33815223; PMCID: PMC8012501. Published March 18, 2021. Accessed June 10, 2024.

CHAPTER 1

1. Hasler C et al. Patella instability in children and adolescents. *EFORT Open Rev.* 2017;1(5):160–166.

2. Bracha H. Freeze, Flight, fight, fright, faint: Adaptationist perspectives on the acute stress response spectrum. *CNS Spectrums.* 2004; 9(9): 679–685.

3. Kozlowska K et al. Fear and the defense cascade: Clinical implications and management. *Harv Rev Psychiatry.* 2015; 23(4):263–287.

4. Ray J. American's stress and worry intensify in 2018. *Gallup World.* April 25, 2019. https://news.gallup.com/poll/249098/americans-stress-worry-anger-intensified-2018.aspx. Accessed September 20, 2023.

5. Baxter M et al. Facing the role of the amygdala in emotional information processing. *PNAS.* 2012;109(52):21180–21181.

6. Bracha H. Freeze, flight, fight, fright, faint: Adaptationist perspectives on acute stress response spectrum. *CNS Spectrums.* 2004; 9(9): 679–685.

7. McEwen BS. Neurobiological and systemic effects of chronic stress. *Chronic Stress.* 2017;1:2470547017692328.

8. Vlachakis C et al. Human emotions on the onset of cardiovascular and small vessel related diseases. *In Vivo.* 2018;32(4):859–870.

9. Morey JN et al. Current directions in stress and human immune function. *Curr Opin Psychol.* 2015;5:13–17.

10. American Heart Association. Inflammation and heart disease. Updated July 31, 2015. https://www.heart.org/en/health-topics/consumer-healthcare/what-is-cardiovascular-disease/inflammation-and-heart-disease Accessed September 15, 2023.

11. Kalmoe MC et al. Physician suicide: A call to action. *Mo Med.* 2019;116(3):211–216.

12. Wild S. (Rep), HR-1667, Dr. Lorna Breen Health Care Provider Protection Act, presented to President on Mar. 11, 2022.

13. Dr. Lorna Breen Healthcare Provider Protection Act, HR1667, 117th Congress, Public Law 117–105. March 18, 2022. https://www.congress.gov/117/plaws/publ105/PLAW-117publ105.pdf. Accessed September 15, 2023.

14. Matias I et al. Occurrence and possible biological role of the endocannabinoid system in the sea squirt ciona intestinalis. *J Neurochem.* 2005 Jun;93(5):1141–56.

15. Devane W et al. Determination and characterization of cannabinoid receptors in rat brain. *Mol Pharmacol.* 1988; 34: 605–613.

16. Devane W et al. Isolation and structure of a brain constituent that binds to the cannabinoid receptor. *Science.* 1992; 258(5090): 1946–1949.

17. Gaoni Y. Isolation and structure of DELTA-tetrahydrocannabinol and other neutral cannabinoids from hashish. *J Am Chem Soc.* 1971;93(1):217–224

18. Di Marzo V et al. The endocannabinoid system and its therapeutic exploitation. *Nat Rev Drug Discov.* 2004; 3: 771–784

19. Russo EB. Clinical endocannabinoid deficiency (CECD): can this concept explain therapeutic benefits of cannabis in migraine, fibromyalgia, irritable bowel syndrome and other treatment-resistant conditions? *Neuro Endocrinol Lett.* 2008 Apr;29(2):192–200.

20. Russo EB. Clinical endocannabinoid deficiency reconsidered: Current research supports the theory in migraine, fibromyalgia, irritable bowel, and other treatment-resistant syndromes. *Cannabis Cannabinoid Res.* 2016 Jul 1;1(1):154–165.

21. Aran A et al. Lower circulating endocannabinoid levels in children with autism spectrum disorder. *Mol Autism.* 2019 Jan 30;10:2.

22. Karhson DS et al. Plasma anandamide concentrations are lower in children with autism spectrum disorder. *Mol Autism.* 2018 Mar 12;9:18.

23. Romigi A et al. Cerebrospinal fluid levels of the endocannabinoid anandamide are reduced in patients with untreated newly diagnosed temporal lobe epilepsy. *Epilepsia.* 2010;51(5):768–772.

CHAPTER 2

1. Mariotti A. The effects of chronic stress on health: new insights into the molecular mechanisms of brain-body communication. *Future Sci OA*. 2015;1(3):FSO23.

2. Warren KR et al. Role of chronic stress and depression in periodontal diseases. *Periodontol* 2000; 64: 127–138.

3. Cohen S et al. Psychological stress and susceptibility to the common cold. *N Engl J Med*. 1991;325(9):606–612.

4. Kopp M et al. Where psychology meets physiology: chronic stress and premature mortality—the Central-Eastern European health paradox, *Brain Research Bulletin*. 2014;62(5) 351–367.

5. Keyes CLM. Chronic physical conditions and aging: Is mental health a potential protective factor? *Ageing International*. 2005; 30: 88–104.

6. HJ Eysenck. Cancer, personality and stress: Prediction and prevention. *Advances in Behaviour Research and Therapy*, 1994;16(3) 167–215.

7. HJ Eysenck. Cancer, personality and stress: Prediction and prevention. *Advances in Behaviour Research and Therapy*. 1994;16(3) 167–215.

8. Hwang SW et al. Is looking older than one's actual age a sign of poor health? *J Gen Intern Med*. 2011;26(2):136–141.

9. Cohen S et al. A global measure of perceived stress. *Journal of Health and Social Behavior*. 1983;24: 386–396.

10. Centers for Disease Control and Prevention. Rabies. Updated January 25, 2021. https://www.cdc.gov/rabies/exposure/animals/other.html. Accessed September 20, 2023.

11. Vidal C et al. Social media use and depression in adolescents: a scoping review. *Int Rev Psychiatry*. 2020;32(3):235–253.

12. Perlis RH et al. Association between social media use and self-reported symptoms of depression in US adults. *JAMA Netw Open*. 2021;4(11):e2136113.

13. McKnight-Eily LR et al. Racial and ethnic disparities in the prevalence of stress and worry, mental health conditions, and increased substance use among adults during the COVID-19 pandemic—United States, *MMWR Morb Mortal Wkly Rep* 2021;70:162–166.

14. Wheaton Michael G et al. Is fear of COVID-19 contagious? The effects of emotion contagion and social media use on anxiety in response to the Coronavirus pandemic. *Frontiers in Psychology*, 2011;11.

15. Cannon CE et al. COVID-19, Intimate partner violence, and communication ecologies. *American Behavioral Scientist*. 2021;65(7):992–1013.

16. Su Z, McDonnell D, Wen J et al. Mental health consequences of COVID-19 media coverage: the need for effective crisis communication practices. *Global Health* 2021;17(4).

17. Damian F et al., Global prevalence and burden of depressive and anxiety disorders in 204 countries and territories in 2020 due to the COVID-19 pandemic. *The Lancet*, 2021.

18. Leonard Marie-Jeanne et al. Conspiracy Theories: A public health concern and how to address it, *Frontiers in Psychology*, 2021;12

19. Planas J et al. Trauma Primary Survey, National Library of Medicine. Updated Nov. 7, 2021. Accessed September 20, 2023.

20. Collins P et al. Gender differences in the clinical presentation of heart disease. *Curr Pharm Des.* 2011;17(11):1056–1058.

21. American Heart Association. Heart Attack Symptoms for Women. Updated July 31, 2015. https://www.heart.org/en/health-topics/heart-attack/warning-signs-of -a-heart-attack/heart-attack-symptoms-in-women. Accessed September 20, 2023.

CHAPTER 3

1. Palomba S, et al. Lifestyle and fertility: the influence of stress and quality of life on female fertility. *Reprod Biol Endocrinol.* 2018 Dec 2;16(1):113.

2. Rooney KL, Domar AD. The relationship between stress and infertility. *Dialogues Clin Neurosci.* 2018;20(1):41-47.

3. Kumar P, Sait SF, et al. Ovarian hyperstimulation syndrome. *J Hum Reprod Sci.* 2011 May;4(2):70–5.

4. Aaronson H, Glienke C. A study of the incidence or pregnancy following adoption. *Fertil Steril.* 1963; 14(5): 547–553.

5. Thwaites Annette et. al. How common is natural conception in women who have had a live birth via assisted reproductive technology? Systematic review and meta-analysis, *Human Reproduction.* 2023 August; 38(8): 1590–1600.

6. Jennings LK et. al. Hyperemesis Gravidarum. Updated July 31, 2023. In: StatPearls [Internet]. Treasure Island (FL): StatPearls Publishing; 2023 Jan.

7. Roberts DM et al. Infantile colic. *Am Fam Physician.* 2004 Aug 15;70(4):735–40.

8. Martin CR et al. Review of infant feeding: key features of breast milk and infant formula. *Nutrients.* 2016; 8(5).279.

9. Hanson Lars Å et al. Breast-feeding, infant formulas, and the immune system, *Annals of Allergy, Asthma & Immunology,* 2003; 90(6): 59–63.

10. Luby Joan L et al. Breastfeeding and childhood IQ: the mediating role of gray matter volume, *Journal of the American Academy of Child & Adolescent Psychiatry,* 2016; 55(5): 367–375.

11. Spencer JP. Management of mastitis in breastfeeding women. *Am Fam Physician.* 2008 Sep 15;78(6):727–31.

12. Kair LR et al. Pacifier restriction and exclusive breastfeeding. *Pediatrics.* 2013 Apr;131(4):e1101–7.

13. Val-Laillet D et al. Nonnutritive sucking: one of the major determinants of filial love. *Dev Psychobiol.* 2006 Apr;48(3):220–32.

14. Kair LR et al. Pacifier restriction and exclusive breastfeeding. *Pediatrics.* 2013 Apr;131(4):e1101–7.

15. Limbers CA et al. Physical activity moderates the association between parenting stress and quality of life in working mothers during the COVID-19 pandemic. *Ment Health Phys Act.* 2020 Oct;19:100358.

16. Newman H et al. Mother needs a bigger "helper": A critique of "wine mom" discourse as conformity to hegemonic intensive motherhood. *Sociology Compass*, 2021;15.

17. White A et al. Converging patterns of alcohol use and related outcomes among females and males in the United States, 2002 to 2012. *Alcohol Clin Exp Res.* 2015 Sep;39(9):1712–26.

18. Handley ED et al. Stress-induced drinking in parents of adolescents with externalizing symptomatology: the moderating role of parent social support. *Am J Addict.* 2008 Nov-Dec;17(6):469–77.

19. Lee J, Pellegrini MV. Biochemistry, Telomere and telomerase. Updated December 11, 2022. In: StatPearls [Internet]. Treasure Island (FL): StatPearls Publishing; 2023 Jan.

20. Shammas MA. Telomeres, lifestyle, cancer, and aging. *Curr Opin Clin Nutr Metab Care.* 2011 Jan;14(1):28–34.

21. A Z Pollack et al. Parity associated with telomere length among US reproductive age women. *Human Reproduction*, 2018 April(33)4, 736–744.

22. Barha CK et al. Number of children and telomere length in women: a prospective, longitudinal evaluation. *PLOS ONE* 2016: 11(1): e0146424.

23. Fagan Erin MPH et al. Telomere length is longer in women with late maternal age. *Menopause,* May 2017, 24(5):p 497–501, May 2017.

24. MedlinePlus [Internet]. Bethesda (MD): National Library of Medicine (US). Updated June 24, 2020. Postpartum depression; [reviewed 2022 July 28; cited 2024 Jan. 8]. Available from: https://medlineplus.gov/article/007215.htm.

25. Getahun D et al. Trends in postpartum depression by race/ethnicity and pre-pregnancy body mass index, *AJOG*, Jan. 2023, 228(1), supplement, s122–s123.

26. Lee YL et al. Association of postpartum depression with maternal suicide: A nationwide population-based study. *Int J Environ Res Public Health.* 2022 Apr 23;19(9):5118.

27. Admon LK et al. Trends in suicidality 1 year before and after birth among commercially insured childbearing individuals in the United States, 2006–2017. *JAMA Psychiatry.* 2021 Feb 1;78(2):171–176.

28. Deligiannidis KM et al. Effect of zuranolone vs placebo in postpartum depression: A randomized clinical trial. *JAMA Psychiatry.* 2021;78(9):951–959.

CHAPTER 4

1. Association of American Medical Colleges. Diversity in Medicine: Facts and Figures 2019. https://www.aamc.org/data-reports/workforce/data/figure-12-percentage-us-medical-school-graduates-sex-academic-years-1980-1981-through-2018-2019. Published August 16, 2019. Accessed July 15, 2024.

2. Halpern J., et. al. Women in Urology Residency, 1978-2013: A Critical Look at Gender Representation in Our Specialty. *Urology.* 2016, 92: 20-25.

3. MedlinePlus [Internet]. Bethesda (MD): National Library of Medicine (US). Updated June 24, 2020. Vacuum erectile devices for erection problems; [updated

2023 Sept 20; reviewed 2022 Jan. 17; cited 2024 Jan. 8]. Available from: https://medlineplus.gov/ency/patientinstructions/000985.htm.

4. Mahapatra S et al. Neuroblastoma. Updated July 10, 2023. In: StatPearls [Internet]. Treasure Island (FL): StatPearls Publishing; 2023 Jan.

5. NCADV [Internet]. Austin (TX). Statistics; [cited 2024 Jan. 8]. Available from: https://ncadv.org/statistics.

6. Blome A et al. Pitfalls of extensive documentation in the emergency department. *Ochsner J.* 2020 Fall;20(3):299–302.

7. These 6 physician specialties have the most burnout. American Medical Association. https://www.ama-assn.org/practice-management/physician-health/these-6-physician-specialties-have-most-burnout. Published January 26, 2023. Accessed July 8, 2024.

8. 2022 Fall applicant, matriculant, and enrollment data tables, Association of American Medical Colleges, 2022, Oct. 31.

9. Bickel J. Women in academic medicine. *J Am Med Womens Assoc* (1972). 2000 Winter;55(1):10-2, 19.

10. Mangurian C et al. What's holding women in medicine back from leadership, *Harvard Business Review*, 2018, Nov. 07.

11. Lallukka T et al. Workplace bullying and subsequent psychotropic medication: a cohort study with register linkages, *BMJ Open* 2012;2:e001660.

12. Kivimäki M, Kawachi I. Work stress as a risk factor for cardiovascular disease. *Curr Cardiol Rep.* 2015 Sep;17(9):630.

13. Kubzansky LD et al.. Going to the heart of the matter: do negative emotions cause coronary heart disease? *J Psychosom Res.* 2000 Apr-May;48(4–5):323–37.

14. Vlachakis C et al. Human emotions on the onset of cardiovascular and small vessel related diseases. *In Vivo.* 2018 Jul-Aug;32(4):859–870.

CHAPTER 5

1. Hwang SW et al. Is looking older than one's actual age a sign of poor health? *J Gen Intern Med.* 2011 Feb;26(2):136–41.

2. National Center for Chronic Disease Prevention and Health Promotion. *Centers for Disease Control and Prevention*, (online) https://www.cdc.gov/chronicdisease/index.htm. May 8, 2023.

3. Cleveland Clinic. *Cosmetic Surgery & Skincare*, https://my.clevelandclinic.org/health/articles/11007-cosmetic-surgery-and-skincare. June 28, 2021.

4. Fabi S et al. Facial Aesthetic Priorities and Concerns: A Physician and Patient Perception Global Survey. *Aesthet Surg J.* 2022 Mar 15;42(4):NP218-NP229.

5. Franzblau LE et al. Impact of medical tourism on cosmetic surgery in the United States. *Plast Reconstr Surg Glob Open.* 2013 Nov 7;1(7):e63.

6. Wen N. Direct and indirect effects of mediated celebrity on young people's attitudes toward cosmetic surgery, 2013. Doctoral thesis, Nanyang Technological University, Singapore.

7. Feusner J, et. al. The pathophysiology of body dysmorphic disorder, *Body Image*, 2008(5)3–12.

8. Laughter MR et al. Psychology of aesthetics: Beauty, social media, and body dysmorphic disorder. *Clin Dermatol*. 2023 Jan-Feb;41(1):28–32.

9. Buttorff C et al. *Multiple Chronic Conditions in the United States*, RAND Corporation, TL-221-PFCD, 2017. As of February 16, 2024.

10. Ross R et al. Waist circumference as a vital sign in clinical practice: a Consensus Statement from the IAS and ICCR Working Group on Visceral Obesity. *Nat Rev Endocrinol*. 2020 Mar;16(3):177–189.

11. American Council on Exercise, Exercise and Cellulite, *Fit Facts*, 2009, www.acefitness.org/GetFit.

12. Speakman JR, Selman C. Physical activity and resting metabolic rate. *Proceedings of the Nutrition Society*. 2003;62(3):621-634.

13. Grogan S et al. Smoking to stay thin or giving up to save face? Young men and women talk about appearance concerns and smoking, *British Journal of Health Psychology*, 2011 Jan;14(1):175–186.

14. Whitefield-Madrano A. How my mirror fast landed me on the Today Show—and my thighs on national television. Updated December 6, 2017. *Huffpost*, 2012 Aug 28.

15. Dreisbach S. Shocking body-image news: 97% of women will be cruel to their bodies today, *Glamour*, 2011. Online.

16. Diller V. The psychology behind a "good hair day," *Huffpost-Blog*, January 31, 2012. Online.

17. Vinocur L. Health from the outside-in, *Huffpost-Blog*, April 2, 2012. Online.

18. Suissa, A. Addiction to Cosmetic Surgery: Representations and Medicalization of the Body. *Int J Ment Health Addiction* 2008; 6: 619-630

19. Moore CA et al. Anorexia Nervosa. Updated August 28, 2023. In: StatPearls [Internet]. Treasure Island (FL): StatPearls Publishing; 2024 Jan. Available from: https://www.ncbi.nlm.nih.gov/books/NBK459148/

20. Hosseini SA et al. Body Image Distortion. [Updated 2023 Sep 4]. In: StatPearls [Internet]. Treasure Island (FL): StatPearls Publishing; 2024 Jan. Available from: https://www.ncbi.nlm.nih.gov/books/NBK546582/

21. Fryar C., et. al. Prevalence of overweight, obesity, and severe obesity among adults aged 20 and over: United States, 1960–1962 through 2017–2018. NCHS Health E-Stats, Centers for Disease Control and Prevention. 2020. https://www.cdc.gov/nchs/data/hestat/obesity-adult-17-18/obesity-adult.htm Updated February 8, 2021. Accessed July 17, 2024

22. Benavidez GA, Zahnd WE, Hung P, Eberth JM. Chronic Disease Prevalence in the US: Sociodemographic and Geographic Variations by Zip Code Tabulation Area. Prev Chronic Dis 2024;21:230267. DOI: http://dx.doi.org/10.5888/pcd21.230267.

23. Baumeister RF et al. (2003). Does high self-esteem cause better performance, interpersonal success, happiness, or healthier lifestyles? *Psychological Science in the Public Interest*, 4(1), 1–44.

24. Ludman EJ et al. Improving confidence for self care in patients with depression and chronic illnesses. *Behav Med*. 2013;39(1):1–6.

25. Hecht D. The neural basis of optimism and pessimism. *Exp Neurobiol.* 2013 Sep;22(3):173–99.

26. Rozanski A et al. Association of optimism with cardiovascular events and all-cause mortality: A systematic review and meta-analysis. *JAMA Netw Open.* 2019;2(9):e1912200.

27. Lemola S et al. Optimism and self-esteem are related to sleep. Results from a large community-based sample. *Int J Behav Med.* 2013 Dec;20(4):567–71.

28. Neff KD. Self-Compassion, Self-Esteem, and Well-Being. Social and *Personality Psychology Compass*, 2011. 5: 1–12.

CHAPTER 6

1. Tsugawa Y et al. Comparison of Hospital Mortality and Readmission Rates for Medicare Patients Treated by Male vs Female Physicians. *JAMA Intern Med.* 2017;177(2):206–213.

2. Roter DL et al. Physician Gender Effects in Medical Communication: A Meta-analytic Review. *JAMA.* 2002;288(6):756–764.

3. Wallis CJD et al. Surgeon Sex and Long-Term Postoperative Outcomes Among Patients Undergoing Common Surgeries. *JAMA Surg.* 2023;158(11):1185–1194.

4. Heiser S. The majority of U.S. medical students are women, new data show-press release, *Association of American Medical Colleges* (online) 9 Dec 2019.

5. Mangurian C et. al. What's Holding Women in Medicine Back from Leadership. *HBR.* https://hbr.org/2018/06/whats-holding-women-in-medicine-back -from-leadership#:~:text=Yetpercent20overallpercent20womenpercent20makep ercent20up,thepercent20resourcespercent20atpercent20medicalpercent20centers. Updated November 7, 2018. Accessed July 27, 2024.

6. Conway CA et. al. 2008 Evidence for adaptive design in human gaze prefer-ence, *Proc. R. Soc. B.*27563–69.

7. Davis JI et al. How does facial feedback modulate emotional experience? *J Res Pers.* 2009 Oct 1;43(5):822–829.

8. Lewis MB et al. Botulinum toxin cosmetic therapy correlates with a more positive mood. *J Cosmet Dermatol.* 2009 Mar;8(1):24–6.

9. Alam M et al. Botulinum toxin and the facial feedback hypothesis: can look-ing better make you feel happier? *J Am Acad Dermatol.* 2008 Jun;58(6):1061–72.

10. Lewis MB. The interactions between botulinum-toxin-based facial treatments and embodied emotions. *Sci Rep.* 2018 Oct 3;8(1):14720.

11. Robins RW et. al. Global self-esteem across the life span. *Psychol. Aging,* 2002; 17(3):423–434.

12. Antonucci TC et al. The relationship between self-esteem and physical health in a family practice population. *Fam Pract Res J.* 1989 Fall-Winter;9(1):65–72.

13. Lamers SM et al. The impact of emotional well-being on long-term recovery and survival in physical illness: a meta-analysis. *J Behav Med.* 2012 Oct;35(5):538–47.

14. Hecht D. The neural basis of optimism and pessimism. *Exp Neurobiol.* 2013 Sep;22(3):173–99.

15. Eagleson C et al. The power of positive thinking: Pathological worry is reduced by thought replacement in Generalized Anxiety Disorder. *Behav Res Ther.* 2016 Mar;78:13–8.

16. vanOyen-Witvliet C et al. Granting forgiveness or harboring grudges: implications for emotion, physiology, and health. *Psychol Sci.* 2001 Mar;12(2):117–23.

17. Williams J et al. Anger proneness predicts coronary heart disease risk, *Circulation* (American Heart Association), 2 May 2000(101)17:2034–2039.

18. Chang PP et al. Anger in young men and subsequent premature cardiovascular disease: the precursors study. *Arch Intern Med.* 2002 Apr 22;162(8):901–6.

19. Taggart P et al. Anger, emotion, and arrhythmias: from brain to heart. *Front Physiol.* 2011 Oct 19;2:67..

20. Lampert R. Anger and ventricular arrhythmias. *Curr Opin Cardiol.* 2010 Jan;25(1):46–52.

21. Ohira T et al. Impact of anger expression on blood pressure levels in white-color workers with low-coping behavior. *Environ Health Prev Med.* 2000 Apr;5(1):37–42.

22. Herrero N et al. What happens when we get angry? Hormonal, cardiovascular and asymmetrical brain responses. *Horm Behav.* 2010 Mar;57(3):276–83.

23. Alfaddagh A et al. Inflammation and cardiovascular disease: From mechanisms to therapeutics. *Am J Prev Cardiol.* 2020 Nov 21;4:100130.

24. Morey JN et al. Current Directions in Stress and Human Immune Function. *Curr Opin Psychol.* 2015 Oct 1;5:13–17.

25. Thoma MV et al. The effect of music on the human stress response. *PLoS One.* 2013 Aug 5;8(8):e70156.

26. Adiasto K et al. Music listening and stress recovery in healthy individuals: A systematic review with meta-analysis of experimental studies. *PLoS One.* 2022 Jun 17;17(6):e0270031.

27. Miller M et al. Divergent effects of joyful and anxiety-provoking music on endothelial vasoreactivity. *Psychosom Med.* 2010 May;72(4):354–6.

28. Jäncke L. Music, memory and emotion. *J Biol.* 2008 Aug 8;7(6):21.

29. Laird KT et. al. Conscious dance: Perceived benefits and psychological well-being of participants. *Comp. Ther. Clin. Pract.* 2021;44.

30. Trivedi G et al. Humming (simple bhramari pranayama) as a stress buster: a holter-based study to analyze heart rate variability (HRV) parameters during bhramari, physical activity, emotional stress, and sleep. *Cureus.* 2023 Apr 13;15(4):e37527.

31. Lo Martire V et al. Stress & sleep: A relationship lasting a lifetime, *Neurosci. Biobehav. Rev.* 2020(11)65–77

32. American Psychological Association. Sleep and Stress. Published 2013. https://www.apa.org/news/press/releases/stress/2013/sleep#:~:text=Adultspercent25 20whopercent2520sleeppercent2520fewerpercent2520than,6.2percent2520hours). Accessed February 17, 2024.

33. National Heart, Lung, and Blood Institute (online). What are sleep deprivation and deficiency? https://www.nhlbi.nih.gov/health/sleep-deprivation, 24 Mar 2022. Accessed March 8, 2024.

34. Institute of Medicine (US) Committee on Sleep Medicine and Research; Colten HR, Altevogt BM, editors. Sleep Disorders and Sleep Deprivation: An Unmet Public Health Problem. Washington (DC): National Academies Press (US); 2006. 4, Functional and Economic Impact of Sleep Loss and Sleep-Related Disorders. Available from: https://www.ncbi.nlm.nih.gov/books/NBK19958/.

35. Eugene AR et al. The Neuroprotective Aspects of Sleep. *MEDtube Sci.* 2015 Mar;3(1):35–40.

36. Besedovsky L et al. Sleep and immune function. *Pflugers Arch.* 2012 Jan;463(1):121–37.

37. Khan MS et al. The effects of insomnia and sleep loss on cardiovascular disease. *Sleep Med Clin.* 2017 Jun;12(2):167–177.

38. Cooper CB et al. Sleep deprivation and obesity in adults: a brief narrative review. *BMJ Open Sport Exerc Med.* 2018 Oct 4;4(1):e000392.

39. Walker M; Kerkhof Gerard A and P.A. van Dongen Hans, editors. Sleep, memory and emotion, *Elsevier: Prog. Brain Res.,* 2010(185)49–68.

40. Louie D et al. The laughter prescription: a tool for lifestyle medicine. *Am J Lifestyle Med.* 2016 Jun 23;10(4):262–267.

41. Seaward BL. Humor's healing potential. *Health Prog.* 1992 Apr;73(3):66–70.

42. Hirosaki M et al. Effects of a laughter and exercise program on physiological and psychological health among community-dwelling elderly in Japan: randomized controlled trial. *Geriatr Gerontol Int.* 2013 Jan;13(1):152–60.

43. Law M et al. A comparison of the cardiovascular effects of simulated and spontaneous laughter. *Complement. Ther. Med.* 2018(37)103–109

44. Yim J. Therapeutic benefits of laughter in mental health: a theoretical review. *Tohoku J Exp Med.* 2016 Jul;239(3):243–9.

45. Wild B et al. Neural correlates of laughter and humour, *Brain,* 2003(126)10:2121–2138.

46. Manninen S et al. Social laughter triggers endogenous opioid release in humans. *J Neurosci.* 2017 Jun 21;37(25):6125–6131.

47. Bennett MP et al. The effect of mirthful laughter on stress and natural killer cell activity. *Altern Ther Health Med.* 2003 Mar-Apr;9(2):38–45.

48. Bast ES et al. Laugh away the fat? Therapeutic humor in the control of stress-induced emotional eating. *Rambam Maimonides Med J.* 2014 Jan 21;5(1):e0007.

49. Rogers C et al. Home and the extended-self: Exploring associations between clutter and wellbeing. *J. Environ. Psychol.* 2021(73).

50. Ferrari JR et al. Delaying disposing: examining the relationship between procrastination and clutter across generations. *Curr Psychol* 37, 426–431 (2018).

51. McMains S et al. Interactions of top-down and bottom-up mechanisms in human visual cortex. *J Neurosci.* 2011 Jan 12;31(2):587–97.

52. Ferrari J et al. The negative side of office clutter: impact on work-related well-being and job satisfaction. *N. Am. J. Psychol.* 2020(22) 441–454.

53. An S et al. To discard or not to discard: the neural basis of hoarding symptoms in obsessive-compulsive disorder. *Mol Psychiatry* 2009(14)318–331.

54. McMains S et al. Interactions of top-down and bottom-up mechanisms in human visual cortex. *J Neurosci.* 2011 Jan 12;31(2):587–97.

55. Hanley AW et al. Washing dishes to wash the dishes: brief instruction in an informal mindfulness practice. *Mindfulness* 2015(6)1095–1103.

56. Hanley AW et al. Washing dishes to wash the dishes: brief instruction in an informal mindfulness practice. *Mindfulness* 2015(6)1095–1103.

57. Sorrell JM. Tidying up: good for the aging brain. *J Psychosoc Nurs Ment Health Serv.* 2020 Apr 1;58(4):16–18.

58. White MP et al. Spending at least 120 minutes a week in nature is associated with good health and wellbeing. *Sci Rep, 2019*(9) 7730.

59. Kardan O et al. Neighborhood greenspace and health in a large urban center. *Sci Rep, 2015*(5) 11610.

60. Halonen JI et al. Green and blue areas as predictors of overweight and obesity in an 8-year follow-up study. *Obesity (Silver Spring).* 2014 Aug;22(8):1910–7.

61. Astell-Burt T et al. Is neighborhood green space associated with a lower risk of type 2 diabetes? Evidence from 267,072 Australians. *Diabetes Care.* 2014;37(1):197–201.

62. Mitchell RJ et al. Neighborhood environments and socioeconomic inequalities in mental well-being. *Am J Prev Med.* 2015 Jul;49(1):80–4.

63. Gascon M et al. Residential green spaces and mortality: A systematic review. *Environ Int.* 2016 Jan;86:60–7.

64. Hedblom M et al. Reduction of physiological stress by urban green space in a multisensory virtual experiment. *Sci Rep* 2019(9) 10113.

65. Park BJ et al. The physiological effects of Shinrin-yoku (taking in the forest atmosphere or forest bathing): evidence from field experiments in 24 forests across Japan. *Environ Health Prev Med.* 2010 Jan;15(1):18–26.

66. Goto Y et al. Physical and mental effects of bathing: a randomized intervention study. *Evid Based Complement Alternat Med.* 2018 Jun 7;2018:9521086.

67. Goto Y et al. Physical and mental effects of bathing: a randomized intervention study. *Evid Based Complement Alternat Med.* 2018 Jun 7;2018:9521086.

68. Haghayegh S et al. Before-bedtime passive body heating by warm shower or bath to improve sleep: A systematic review and meta-analysis. *Sleep Med Rev.* 2019 Aug;46:124–135.

69. Zhang X et al. Waterscapes for promoting mental health in the general population. *Int J Environ Res Public Health.* 2021 Nov 10;18(22):11792.

70. Holt-Lunstad J et al. Our epidemic of loneliness and isolation, The U.S. Surgeon General's Advisory on the Healing Effects of Social Connection and Community, 2023.

71. Shovestul B et al. Risk factors for loneliness: The high relative importance of age versus other factors. *PLoS One, 2020*, 15(2): e0229087.

72. Weissbourd R et al. Loneliness in America: how the pandemic has deepened an epidemic of loneliness and what we can do about it, Harvard Graduate School of Education (Making Caring Common), 2020.

73. Centers for Disease Control and Prevention (online). Health risks of social isolation and loneliness. 30 Mar 2023. https://www.cdc.gov/emotional-wellbeing/social-connectedness/loneliness.htm. Accessed March 8, 2024.

74. Løseth GE et al. Stress recovery with social support: A dyadic stress and support task. *Psychoneuroendocrinol,* 2022 Dec;146:105949.

75. Sharma A et al. Exercise for mental health. *Prim Care Companion J Clin Psychiatry.* 2006;8(2):106.

76. Yau S-Y et al. Adult hippocampal neurogenesis: A possible way how physical exercise counteracts stress. *Cell Transplant.* 2011;20(1):99–111.

77. Ahmadi MN, Clare PJ, Katzmarzyk PT, *et al.* Vigorous physical activity, incident heart disease, and cancer: how little is enough? *Eur Heart J.* 2022. doi:10.1093/eurheartj/ehac572.

78. Winters C. Short bouts of exercise benefit health, too, *LiveScience (online).* January 13, 2013.

79. Fabel K, et. al. Physical activity and the regulation of neurogenesis in the adult and aging brain. *Neuromol Med* 2008(10)59–66.

80. Alty J, et. al. Exercise and dementia prevention, *Pract. Neurol.* Published Online First: 21 Jan 2020. Accessed March 8, 2024.

81. Law C, et. al. Physical exercise attenuates cognitive decline and reduces behavioural problems in people with mild cognitive impairment and dementia: a systematic review, *J. Physiother.* 2020(66)1:9-18.

82. Hojman, P, et. al. Molecular mechanisms linking exercise to cancer prevention and treatment, *Cell Metab*, 19 Oct 2017(27)1:10-21.

83. Rajarajeswaran, P, et. al. Exercise in cancer, *Indian J Med Paediatr Oncol,* Apr-Jun 2009(30)2

84. Jayedi A, et. al. Central fatness and risk of all cause mortality: systematic review and dose-response meta-analysis of 72 prospective cohort studies, *BMJ,* 2020; 370 :m3324.

85. National Heart, Lung, and Blood Institute (online). Assessing your weight and health risk. https://www.nhlbi.nih.gov/health/educational/lose_wt/risk.htm#:~:text=Evenpercent20apercent20smallpercent20weightpercent20loss,gainpercent20ratherpercent20thanpercent20losepercent20weight. Accessed March 8, 2024.

86. Safron A. What is orgasm? A model of sexual trance and climax via rhythmic entrainment, *Socioaffect Neurosci Psychol*, 2016(6)1.

87. Khajehei M et al. Endorphins, oxytocin, sexuality and romantic relationships: An understudied area. *World J Obstet Gynecol,* 2018; 7(2): 17–23.

88. Klein C et al. Circulating endocannabinoid concentrations and sexual arousal in women. *J Sex Med.* 2012 Jun;9(6):1588–601.

89. Olff M et al. The role of oxytocin in social bonding, stress regulation and mental health: An update on the moderating effects of context and interindividual differences, *Psychoneuroendocrinology*, 2013(38)9:1883–1894.

90. Brody S et al. The post-orgasmic prolactin increase following intercourse is greater than following masturbation and suggests greater satiety. *Biol Psychol.* 2006 Mar;71(3):312–5.

91. Sumioka H et al. Huggable communication medium decreases cortisol levels. *Sci Rep* 2013(3)3034.

92. Eisenbeiss C. et. al. The influence of female sex hormones on skin thickness: evaluation using 20 MHz sonography, *BJD*, 1 Sept 1998(139)3:462–467.

93. Weeks D.Sex for the mature adult: Health, self-esteem and countering ageist stereotypes, *Sexual and Relationship Therapy*, 2002(17)3:231–240.

94. Frappier J et al. Energy expenditure during sexual activity in young health couples, *PLoS One*, 24 Oct 2013, 8(10): e79342.

95. Hall S et al. Sexual activity, erectile dysfunction, and incident cardiovascular events, *Am J Card*, 15 Jan 2015 (105) 2:192–197.

96. Wright H et al. Sex on the brain! Associations between sexual activity and cognitive function in older age, *Age Ageing*, Mar 2016(45)2:313–317.

97. Allen MS. Sexual activity and cognitive decline in older adults. *Arch Sex Behav*, 2018(47): 1711–1719.

98. Bhupathiraju SN et al. Vaginal estrogen use and chronic disease risk in the Nurses' Health Study. *Menopause,* 2018 Dec 17;26(6):603–610.

99. Wong MYC. Considering self-care in High school home economics education with the aid of scoping reviews of mindfulness and cooking and of mindfulness and knitting. *Youth.* 2023; 3(4):1317–1329.

100. Grossman P et al. Mindfulness-based stress reduction and health benefits: A meta-analysis, *J. Psychosom. Res.* 2004(57)1:35–43.

101. Praissman S. Mindfulness-based stress reduction: A literature review and clinician's guide. *J. Am. Acad. Nurse Prac.*, 2008(20): 212–216.

102. Grossman P et al. Mindfulness-based stress reduction and health benefits: A meta-analysis, *J. Psychosom. Res.* 2004(57)1:35–43.

103. Khoury B. Mindfulness-based stress reduction for healthy individuals: A meta-analysis, *J. Psychosom. Res.* 2015(78)6:519–528.

104. Tamlin S, et. al. Everyday creative activity as a path to flourishing, *J. Posit. Psychol.* 2018(13)2:181-189.

105. Farmer N et al. Psychosocial benefits of cooking interventions: A systematic review. *HE&B.* 2018;45(2):167–180.

106. Kochman M et al. Benefits of cooking for mental health, stay away from stress, *Splash Magz*, Mar 2021(1)1.

107. Noda S et al. The effectiveness of intervention with board games: a systematic review. *BioPsychoSocial Med,* 2019(13)22.

108. Desai V et al. Stress-reducing effects of playing a casual video game among undergraduate students, *Trends in Psychol.* 2021(29)563–579.

109. Van Lith T Art therapy in mental health: A systematic review of approaches and practices, *Arts Psychother.* 2016(47)9–22.

110. Kaimal G. et. al., Reduction of Cortisol Levels and Participants' Responses Following Art Making. *Art Ther* (Alex). 2016; 33(2):74–80.

111. Nagasawa M et al Dog's gaze at its owner increases owner's urinary oxytocin during social interaction, *Horm Behav.* 2009(55)3: 434–441.

112. Levine G et.al. Pet ownership and cardiovascular risk, *Circ.* 2013;127:2353–2363.

113. Stanley IH et al. Pet ownership may attenuate loneliness among older adult primary care patients who live alone. *Aging Ment Health.* 2014;18(3):394–9.

114. Beetz A et al. Psychosocial and psychophysiological effects of human-animal interactions: the possible role of oxytocin. *Front. Psychol.* 9 Jul 2012(3)234.

115. Kramer C et al. Dog ownership and survival, *Circulation: Cardiovascular Quality and Outcomes.* 2019;12:e005554.

116. Westgarth C et al. Dog owners are more likely to meet physical activity guidelines than people without a dog: An investigation of the association between dog ownership and physical activity levels in a UK community. *Sci Rep* 2019(9)5704.

CHAPTER 7

1. American Heart Association. Chronic stress can cause heart trouble. Published February 4, 2020. https://www.heart.org/en/news/2020/02/04/chronic-stress-can-cause-heart-trouble#:~:text=Stress percent20may percent20lead percent20to percent20high,cardiovascular percent20events percent2C percent22 percent20Schiffrin percent20said. Accessed July 8, 2024.

2. Letourneau SM, Mitchell SE, Ryan AM. How Providers, Payers, and Community Organizations Can Collaborate to Improve Outcomes for Patients with Complex Needs. *N Engl J Med Catalyst.* Published February 15, 2021. https://www.ncbi.nlm.nih.gov/pmc/articles/PMC7864285/. Accessed July 8, 2024.

3. Khera R, Valero-Elizondo J, Nasir K. Financial Toxicity of Medical Debt: An Underappreciated Driver of Health Inequities. *Lancet.* 2022;399(10334):1047–1048.

4. Thaker P, Han LY, Kamat AA, et al. Chronic Stress Promotes Tumor Growth and Angiogenesis in a Mouse Model of Ovarian Carcinoma. *Cancer Cell.* 2024;36(1):190–204.

5. Babić A, Rendulić K, Buljan M, et al. Stress and Burnout Among Healthcare Workers During the COVID-19 Pandemic. *J Health Soc Sci.* 2021;6(1):25–39.

6. American Public Health Association. The Impacts of Individual and Household Debt on Health and Well-Being. January 7, 2022. https://www.apha.org/Policies-and-Advocacy/Public-Health-Policy-Statements/Policy-Database/2022/01/07/The-Impacts-of-Individual-and-Household-Debt-on-Health-and-Well-Being. Accessed July 20, 2024.

7. Sweetman A, Bradbury K, May C, et al. Exploring the relationships between patient and practitioner characteristics and outcomes in the delivery of community-based support for people with chronic low back pain: a prospective cohort study. *Chiropr Man Therap.* 2015;23:26. https://www.ncbi.nlm.nih.gov/pmc/articles/PMC3667200/.

8. American Psychological Association. Money Stress Weighs on Americans' Health. February 2015. https://www.apa.org/news/press/releases/2015/02/money-stress.

9. Kelly SJ, Ismail M. Stress and Type 2 Diabetes: A Review of How Stress Contributes to the Development of Type 2 Diabetes. *Annu Rev Public Health.* 2015;36:441–462. https://www.ncbi.nlm.nih.gov/pmc/articles/PMC3230928/.

10. Boyce C, Delaney L, Ferguson E, Wood A. Central bank interest rate decisions, household indebtedness, and psychiatric morbidity and distress: Evidence from the UK, *Journal of Affective Disorders*, Volume 234, 2018.

11. Pool LR, Burgard SA, Needham BL, Elliott MR, Langa KM, Mendes de Leon CF. Association of a Negative Wealth Shock With All-Cause Mortality in Middle-aged and Older Adults in the United States. *Soc Sci Med*. 2013;97:239-246. https://www.sciencedirect.com/science/article/abs/pii/S0277953613002839.

12. Dyer O. US Maternal Mortality Hits Highest Level Since 1965, with Black Women Most at Risk. *BMJ*. 2022;376. https://www.ncbi.nlm.nih.gov/pmc/articles/PMC8806009/.

13. Lampert R. Anger and ventricular arrhythmias. *Curr Opin Cardiol*. 2010 Jan;25(1):46-52. doi: 10.1097/HCO.0b013e32833358e8. PMID: 19864944; PMCID: PMC3140423.

14. Momen NC, Plana-Ripoll O, Agerbo E, et al. Association Between Mental Disorders and Subsequent Medical Conditions. *N Engl J Med*. 2020;382(18):1721–1731. https://www.ncbi.nlm.nih.gov/pmc/articles/PMC6175215/.

15. Nolen-Hoeksema S, Hilt LM. Emotion Regulation and Psychopathology. *Behav Ther*. 2020;51(6):834-845. https://www.sciencedirect.com/science/article/abs/pii/S0306460320306870.

16. Jeste DV, Palmer BW, Appelbaum PS, et al. A New Paradigm for Research on the Trajectory of Schizophrenia and Its Modifiable Risk Factors. *JAMA Psychiatry*. 2019;76(9):914–922. https://www.ncbi.nlm.nih.gov/pmc/articles/PMC6799954/.

17. Walker ER, McGee RE, Druss BG. Mortality in Mental Disorders and Global Disease Burden Implications: A Systematic Review and Meta-analysis. *JAMA Psychiatry*. 2015;72(4):334–341. https://www.ncbi.nlm.nih.gov/pmc/articles/PMC5403578/.

18. McGorry PD, Killackey E, Yung A. Early Intervention in Psychosis: Concepts, Evidence and Future Directions. *World Psychiatry*. 2008;7(3):148–156. https://www.ncbi.nlm.nih.gov/pmc/articles/PMC2453310/.

19. Galea S, Merchant RM, Lurie N. The Mental Health Consequences of COVID-19 and Physical Distancing: The Need for Prevention and Early Intervention. *JAMA Intern Med*. 2020;180(6):817–818. https://www.ncbi.nlm.nih.gov/pmc/articles/PMC7283754/.

20. Smith SM, Kosslyn SM. Functional Imaging of Human Memory. *Neuron*. 2023. https://www.cell.com/neuron/abstract/S0896-6273(23)00383-5?_returnURL=https percent3A percent2F percent2Flinkinghub.elsevier.com percent2Fretrieve percent-2Fpii percent2FS0896627323003835 percent3Fshowall percent3Dtrue.

21. Swedo SE, Leonard HL, Garvey M, et al. Pediatric Autoimmune Neuropsychiatric Disorders Associated with Streptococcal Infections (PANDAS). J Child Neurol. 2014;29(9):1153–1167. https://www.ncbi.nlm.nih.gov/pmc/articles/PMC4214609/.

22. Hayes S et al. Am I too fat to be a princess? Examining the effects of popular children's media on young girls' body image. *British J of Develop Psychol*. 2010; 28(2): 413–426.

23. Shisslak C et al. The spectrum of eating disturbances. *Int J Eat Disord*. 1995; 18(3): 209–219.

24. Menon V. Complex Brain Networks: From Connections to Cognition. Neuron. 2020;107(6):1031–1036. https://www.ncbi.nlm.nih.gov/pmc/articles/PMC7538029/. Accessed July 22, 2024.

25. Bonito AJ, Bann CM, Eicheldinger CR, et al. Differential Response to Educational Strategies by Ethnicity and Language Preference: A Longitudinal Analysis of Diabetes Self-Management. *BMC Public Health*. 2014;14:647. https://www.ncbi.nlm.nih.gov/pmc/articles/PMC4241770/.

26. Fishbane S, Pollack VE, Feldman HI, et al. Safety and Efficacy of Ferric Citrate in Patients with Non–Dialysis-Dependent Chronic Kidney Disease. *N Engl J Med*. 2015;372(12):1044–1055. https://www.nejm.org/doi/full/10.1056/NEJMoa1606148.

27. Sharifi-Rad J, Rodrigues CF, Sharopov F, et al. Diet, Lifestyle and Cardiovascular Diseases: Linking Pathophysiology to Cardioprotective Effects of Natural Bioactive Compounds. *Nutrients*. 2020;12(7):1955. https://www.mdpi.com/2072-6643/12/7/1955.

28. Liu J, Feng X, Li J, et al. The Power of Play: The Importance of Play in Physical Activity, Health, and Well-Being. *Front Psychol*. 2020;11:2021. https://www.ncbi.nlm.nih.gov/pmc/articles/PMC7770496/.

29. Yamamoto Y, Takeuchi R, Nakagawa T, et al. The Impact of COVID-19 on Lifestyle Changes, Symptoms, and Psychological Distress in Japanese People. *PLoS One*. 2020;15(12)
. https://www.ncbi.nlm.nih.gov/pmc/articles/PMC7746965/.

30. Thurlow AJ, Zuo Y, Miller A, et al. Environmental Impacts on Health and Wellness: Integrating Science and Policy for Positive Change. *Int J Environ Res Public Health*. 2015;12(10):12836–12846. https://www.ncbi.nlm.nih.gov/pmc/articles/PMC4696435/.

31. Miller ES, Gur RC, Kinney DK, et al. The Role of Genetics in Brain Development and Cognitive Function. *J Neurosci*. 2020;40(48):9239–9246. https://www.ncbi.nlm.nih.gov/pmc/articles/PMC7014832/

32. Kumar A, Smith Z, Yadav R, et al. Advances in Understanding of Cognitive Decline and Brain Aging. *J Gerontol A Biol Sci Med Sci*. 2023;78(4):601–611. https://www.ncbi.nlm.nih.gov/pmc/articles/PMC8954878/.

33. Iizuka K. Is the Use of Artificial Sweeteners Beneficial for Patients with Diabetes Mellitus? The Advantages and Disadvantages of Artificial Sweeteners. Nutrients. 2022 Oct 22;14(21):4446. doi: 10.3390/nu14214446. PMID: 36364710; PMCID: PMC9655943.

34. Park S, Kim H, Song J. Associations Between Dietary Patterns and Mental Health in Korean Adolescents: A Cross-Sectional Study. *BMC Public Health*. 2017;17:417. https://www.ncbi.nlm.nih.gov/pmc/articles/PMC5664675/.

35. Atkinson FS, Foster-Powell K, Brand-Miller JC. International Tables of Glycemic Index and Glycemic Load Values: 2008. *Diabetes Care*. 2008;31(12):2281–2283. https://diabetesjournals.org/care/article/31/12/2281/24911/International-Tables-of-Glycemic-Index-and

36. Nakamura T, Koike H, Ichimura H, et al. Advances in Understanding the Pathophysiology of Diabetic Neuropathy. *J Diabetes Complications*. 2023;47(1):108203. https://www.ncbi.nlm.nih.gov/pmc/articles/PMC9723158/.

37. Liu, A.G., Ford, N.A., Hu, F.B. *et al.* A healthy approach to dietary fats: understanding the science and taking action to reduce consumer confusion. *Nutr J* 2017;**16**: 53. https://doi.org/10.1186/s12937-017-0271-4

38. Unroe KT, Nazir A, Holbein D, et al. The Complexity of Preventing Dementia: The Role of Social Networks. *JAMA Intern Med.* 2016;176(10):1432–1439. https://jamanetwork.com/journals/jamainternalmedicine/article-abstract/2548255.

39. American Heart Association. Dietary Fats. https://www.heart.org/en/healthy-living/healthy-eating/eat-smart/fats/dietary-fats.

40. Gupta R, Kumar A, Sharma R. Role of Physical Activity in the Prevention and Management of Cardiovascular Disease. *J Cardiovasc Med.* 2023;48(2):141–151. https://www.ncbi.nlm.nih.gov/pmc/articles/PMC9963093/.

41. Grundy SM, Cleeman JI, Daniels SR, et al. Diagnosis and Management of the Metabolic Syndrome: An American Heart Association/National Heart, Lung, and Blood Institute Scientific Statement. Circulation. 2005;112(17):2735–2752. https://www.ahajournals.org/doi/full/10.1161/CIRCULATIONAHA.106.176158.

42. McGee DL. Role of Stress in the Pathogenesis of Cardiovascular Disease. *Am J Cardiol.* 2023;32(4):431–439. https://www.ncbi.nlm.nih.gov/pmc/articles/PMC6466433/.

43. Institute of Medicine (US) Committee on Sleep Medicine and Research; Colten HR, Altevogt BM, editors. Sleep Disorders and Sleep Deprivation: An Unmet Public Health Problem. Washington (DC): National Academies Press (US); 2006. https://www.ncbi.nlm.nih.gov/books/NBK298903/. Accessed March 30, 2024.

44. Center for Economic and Policy Research. Again, the U.S. is a No-Vacation Nation. https://cepr.net/press-release/again-the-us-is-a-no-vacation-nation/.

45. U.S. Bureau of Labor Statistics. Paid Vacations. https://www.bls.gov/ebs/factsheets/paid-vacations.htm.

46. Pew Research Center. More Than 4 in 10 U.S. Workers Don't Take All Their Paid Time Off. https://www.pewresearch.org/short-reads/2023/08/10/more-than-4-in-10-u-s-workers-dont-take-all-their-paid-time-off/#:~:text=More percent-20than percent204 percent20in percent2010,all percent20their percent20paid percent-20time percent20off&text=Some percent2046 percent25 percent20of percent20U.S. percent20workers,recent percent20Pew percent20Research percent20Center percent20survey.

47. Harvard Business Review. How Taking a Vacation Improves Your Well-Being. https://hbr.org/2023/07/how-taking-a-vacation-improves-your-well-being.

48. Kanai A. "Karoshi" (Work to death) in Japan, working to live or living to work. *J Bus Ethics.* 2009; 84(2): 209–216.

49. Kivimäki M and Kawachi I. Work Stress as a Risk Factor for Cardiovascular Disease. *Curr Cardiol Rep.* 2015; (9):630. doi: 10.1007/s11886-015-0630-8. PMID: 26238744; PMCID: PMC4523692.

50. Wang PS, Aguilar-Gaxiola S, Alonso J, et al. Use of Mental Health Services for Anxiety, Mood, and Substance Disorders in the United States and Ontario. https://www.ncbi.nlm.nih.gov/pmc/articles/PMC5891372/

51. Lemaire JB, Wallace JE. Burnout among Physicians. https://www.ncbi.nlm.nih.gov/pmc/articles/PMC5800229/.

52. Gallup. The World's Trillion-Dollar Workplace Problem. https://www.gallup.com/workplace/393497/world-trillion-workplace-problem.aspx

53. American Institute of Stress. Workplace Stress. https://www.stress.org/workplace-stress#:~:text=According percent20to percent20one percent20survey percent2C percent2080,stress percent20particularly percent20leads percent20to percent20burnout.

54. Wall Street Journal. Worker Burnout, Resignations, and Pandemic Stress. Available at: https://www.wsj.com/articles/worker-burnout-resignations-pandemic-stress--11640099198.

55. Corporate Wellness Magazine. Workplace Stress: The Silent Killer of Employee Health & Productivity. https://www.corporatewellnessmagazine.com/article/workplace-stress-silent-killer-employee-health-productivity#

56. PR Newswire. Five Reasons to Make Regular Vacations a Top New Year's Resolution. https://www.prnewswire.com/news-releases/five-reasons-to-make-regular-vacations-a-top-new-years-resolution-300014163.html.

57. Capitanio U, Jeldres C, Perrotte P, Isbarn H, Shariat SF, Zini L, et al. The Use of Ciclosporin in Combination with Low Dose Steroids for the Prevention of Renal Transplant Rejection: A Meta-analysis of Randomized Controlled Trials. *Urol Res.* 2003;31(5):317–322. https://link.springer.com/article/10.1007/s00240-003-0359-5.

58. Kelly SJ, Ismail M. Stress and Type 2 Diabetes: A Review of How Stress Contributes to the Development of Type 2 Diabetes. *Annu Rev Public Health.* 2015;36:441–462. https://www.ncbi.nlm.nih.gov/pmc/articles/PMC3662135/.

59. Dyer O. US Maternal Mortality Hits Highest Level Since 1965, with Black Women Most at Risk. BMJ. 2022;376. https://www.ncbi.nlm.nih.gov/pmc/articles/PMC8733151/.

60. Misra DP, Lager J, Foster HW. The Association Between Maternal Weight Gain and Preterm Delivery: A Review. Am J Perinatol. 2009;26(9):729–734. https://www.ncbi.nlm.nih.gov/pmc/articles/PMC2863117/.

61. Durko A et al. Family and Relationship Benefits of Travel Experiences: A Literature Review. *J Travel Res.* 2013;52(6): 720–730.

CHAPTER 8

1. Yegorov YE et al. The Link between Chronic Stress and Accelerated Aging. *Biomedicines.* 2020 Jul 7;8(7):198.

2. Hwang SW et al. Is looking older than one's actual age a sign of poor health? *J Gen Intern Med.* 2011 Feb;26(2):136–141.

3. Chen Y. Brain-skin connection: stress, inflammation and skin aging. *Inflamm Allergy Drug Targets.* 2014;13(3):177–190.

4. Epel E et al. Accelerated telomere shortening in response to life stress, *PNAS.* Dec 2004, 101 (49) 17312–17315.

5. Proctor & Gamble. New study conducted at Yale University concludes that "bad hair days" affect more than your appearance. Jan 26, 2000. https://www.super-hair.net/yale-hair.html. Accessed May 27, 2024.

6. MacBride Elizabeth. Researchers: A Few Bad Hair Days Can Change Your Life, *Stanford Business*, April 11, 2014, https://www.gsb.stanford.edu/insights/researchers-few-bad-hair-days-can-change-your-life

7. Godoy-Izquierdo D et al. Body Satisfaction, Weight Stigma, Positivity, and Happiness among Spanish Adults with Overweight and Obesity. *Int J Environ Res Public Health*. 2020 Jun 12;17(12):4186.

8. Aniulis E et al. The Real Ideal: Misestimation of Body Mass Index, *Frontiers in Global Women's Health*, Vol. 3, 2022. https://www.frontiersin.org/articles/10.3389/fgwh.2022.756119

9. Lu H et al. The hippocampus underlies the association between self-esteem and physical health. November 20, 2018. *Sci Rep* 2018; 8: 17141. Accessed April 5, 2024. https://doi.org/10.1038/s41598-018-34793-x

10. Cao C et al. Diet and Skin Aging-From the Perspective of Food Nutrition. *Nutrients*. 2020 Mar 24;12(3):870.

11. Contreras RE et al. Physiological and Epigenetic Features of Yoyo Dieting and Weight Control. *Front Genet*. 2019 Dec 11;10:1015.

12. Synnot A. Those weight loss drugs may do a number on your face, *New York Times*, January 23, 2023. https://www.nytimes.com/2023/01/24/style/ozempic-weight-loss-drugs-aging.html. Accessed May 27, 2024.

13. Mekić S et al. A healthy diet in women is associated with less facial wrinkles in a large Dutch population-based cohort, *JAAD*, published May 2019, Vol. 80, Issue 5.

14. Schagen SK et al. Discovering the link between nutrition and skin aging. *Dermatoendocrinol*. 2012 Jul 1;4(3):298–307.

15. Guyuron B et al. Factors Contributing to the Facial Aging of Identical Twins. *Plastic and Reconstructive Surgery* 123(4):p 1321–1331, April 2009.

16. Piwowarska J et al. Serum cortisol concentration in patients with major depression after treatment with fluoxetine. *Psychiatry Res*. 2012;198(3): 407–11.

17. Patel S et al. Anti-inflammatory properties of commonly used psychiatric drugs. January 10, 2023. *Front Neurosci*. 2023 Jan 10;16:1039379. Accessed April 7, 2024.

18. Agrawal R et al. The skin and inflamm-aging. November 2, 2023. *Biology (Base)l* 2023 Nov 2;12(11):1396. Accessed April 6, 2024.

19. Chen Y et al. Brain-skin connection: stress, inflammation and skin aging. *Inflamm Allergy Drug Targets*. 2014;13(3):177–190.

20. Depression, National Institute of Mental Health, National Institute of Mental Health. https://www.nimh.nih.gov/health/topics/depression. Accessed May 27, 2024.

21. Pan A et al. Depression and Incident Stroke in Women, *Stroke*, Aug 2011.

22. Kwapong Y et al. Association of depression and poor mental health with cardiovascular disease and suboptimal cardiovascular health among young adults in the United States. 23 Jan 2023. *JAHA*.

23. Patterson S et al. Depression and anxiety are associated with cardiovascular health in young adults, *JAHA*, 19 Dec 2022;11:e027610.

24. Centers for Disease Control and Prevention. Updated November 2, 2022. *Suicide Prevention: Risk and Protective Factors*. https://www.hhs.gov/answers/mental

-health-and-substance-abuse/does-depression-increase-risk-of-suicide/index.html. Accessed April 6, 2024.

25. Call 988. *About.* https://988helpline.org.

26. American Heart Association. *Go Red for Women.* https://www.goredfor-women.org/en/. Accessed May 27, 2024.

27. Centers for Disease Control and Prevention. *About Women and Heart Disease.* https://www.cdc.gov/heartdisease/women.htm. Accessed May 27, 2024.

28. Woodward M. Cardiovascular Disease and the Female Disadvantage. *Int J Environ Res Public Health.* 2019 Apr 1;16(7):1165.

29. Chen A. Women die more from heart attacks than men—unless the ER doc is female. August 6, 2018. *Scientific American,* https://www.scientificamerican.com/article/women-die-more-from-heart-attacks-than-men-mdash-unless-the-er-doc-is-female/ Accessed April1, 2024.

30. Tsugawa Y, Jena AB, Figueroa JF, Orav EJ, Blumenthal DM, Jha AK. Comparison of Hospital Mortality and Readmission Rates for Medicare Patients Treated by Male vs Female Physicians. *JAMA Intern Med.* 2017;177(2):206–213.

31. Roter DL, Hall JA, Aoki Y. Physician Gender Effects in Medical Communication: A Meta-analytic Review. *JAMA.* 2002;288(6):756–764.

32. Baumhäkel M, Müller U, Böhm M. Influence of gender of physicians and patients on guideline-recommended treatment of chronic heart failure in a cross-sectional study. *Eur J Heart Fail.* 2009 Mar;11(3):299-303.

33. Frank E, Harvey LK. Prevention advice rates of women and men physicians. *Arch Fam Med.* 1996 Apr;5(4):215–9.

34. Redberg RF, Parks AL, Rubin JB. Persistent Gender Pay Gaps in Medicine: What Is Good for the Goose Is Better for the Gander's Paycheck. *JAMA Intern Med.* 2021;181(9):1164. doi:10.1001/jamainternmed.2021.3470

35. American Cancer Society. *Cancer Prevention & Early Detection Facts & Figures 2019–2020.* Published 2019. https://www.cancer.org/content/dam/cancer-org/research/cancer-facts-and-statistics/cancer-prevention-and-early-detection-facts-and-figures/cancer-prevention-and-early-detection-facts-and-figures-2019-2020.pdf. Accessed May 27, 2024.

36. Anand P et al. Cancer is a preventable disease that requires major lifestyle changes. *Pharm Res.* 2008;25(9):2097–116.

37. American Heart Association. Research Adds to Knowledge About Heart Disease and Stroke in Women of All Ages. February 27, 2024. https://newsroom.heart.org/news/research-adds-to-knowledge-about-heart-disease-and-stroke-in-women-of-all-ages#:~:text=Cardiovascular percent20disease percent20kills percent20more percent20women,U.S. percent20have percent20good percent20heart percent20health. Accessed May 27, 2024.

38. Ubrich R et al. Sex differences in long-term mortality among acute myocardial infarction patients: results from the ISAR-RISK and ART studies. October 20, 2017. *PLoS One.* 2017;12(10):e0186783. Accessed April 6, 2024.

39. Elder P et al. Identification of female-specific risk enhancers throughout the lifespan of women to improve cardiovascular disease prevention June 6, 2020. *Am J Prev Cardiol.* 2020 Jun 6;2:100028. Accessed April 6, 2024.

40. Prescott E et al. Smoking and risk of myocardial infarction in women and men: longitudinal population study. April 4, 1998. *BMJ.* 1998 Apr 4;316(7137):1043–7. Accessed April 7, 2024.

41. Gaggin H et al. Gender difference in cardiovascular disease: women are less likely to be prescribed certain heart medications, *Harvard Health Publishing.* October 15, 2020. https://www.health.harvard.edu/blog/gender-differences-in-cardio-vascular-disease-women-are-less-likely-to-be-prescribed-certain-heart-medications -2020071620553. Accessed 27 May 2024.

42. Liu J., et.al. Age-Stratified Sex Disparities in Care and Outcomes in Patients With ST-Elevation Myocardial Infarction. *Am J Med.* 2020;133(11):1293-1301.

43. Martinez-Nadal G et al. An analysis based on sex & gender in the chest pain unit of an emergency department during the last 12 years, *European Heart Journal. Acute Cardiovascular Care,* Volume 10, Issue Supplement 1, April 2021. Accessed 27 May 2024.

44. Zhao M et al. Sex Differences in Cardiovascular Medication Prescription in Primary Care: A Systematic Review and Meta-Analysis. June 20, 2020. *J Am Heart Assoc.* 2020 Jun 2;9(11):e014742. Accessed April 19, 2024.

45. Kochanek, KD et al. (2016). Deaths: final data for 2014. National vital statistics reports: from the Centers for Disease Control and Prevention, National Center for Health Statistics, National Vital Statistics System, 65(4), 1–122.

46. Maas A et al. Gender differences in coronary heart disease. *Neth Heart J.* 2010 Dec;18(12):598–602.

47. Keteepe-Arachi T et al. Cardiovascular Disease in Women: Understanding Symptoms and Risk Factors. *Eur Cardiol.* 2017; 1(1): 10–13.

48. Ross R et al. Waist circumference as a vital sign in clinical practice: a Consensus Statement from the IAS and ICCR Working Group on Visceral Obesity. *Nat Rev Endocrinol.* 2020; 16(3): 177–189.

49. Ernster V. The epidemiology of lung cancer in women. *Ann Epidemiol.* 1994; 4(2): 102–110.

50. Islami F et al. Global trends of lung cancer mortality and smoking prevalence. *Transl Lung Cancer Res.* 2015; 4(4): 327–338.

51. Anand P et al. Cancer is a preventable disease that requires major lifestyle changes. *Pharm Res.* 2008; 25(9): 2097–2116.

52. Charde S et al.. Human papillomavirus prevention by vaccination: a review article. October 2011. *Cureus.* 2022 Oct 7;14(10):e30037. Accessed April 20, 2024.

53. U.S. Preventive Services Task Force. Breast Cancer: Screening. April 30, 2024.
https://www.uspreventiveservicestaskforce.org/uspstf/recommendation/breast -cancer-screening.

54. Bloomfield H et al. Evidence brief: role of the annual comprehensive physical examination in the asymptomatic adult [Internet]. Washington (DC): Department of Veterans Affairs (US); 2011 Oct. https://www.ncbi.nlm.nih.gov/books/ NBK82767/.

55. Oboler S et al. Public expectations and attitudes for annual physical examinations and testing, *Ann Intern Med.2002;136:652–659. [Epub 7 May 2002].*

56. U.S. Department of Health and Human Services. About the Affordable Care Act. Reviewed March 17, 2022. https://www.hhs.gov/healthcare/about-the-aca/index.html#:~:text=The percent2520Patient percent2520Protection percent2520and percent2520Affordable,insurance percent2520available percent2520to percent-2520more percent2520people. Accessed May 27, 2024.

57. Berry T et al. Women's perceptions of heart disease and breast cancer and the association with media representations of the diseases. December 2, 2016. *J Public Health (Oxf)*. 2016 Dec 2;38(4):e496-e503. Accessed April 20, 2024.

58. Hwang ES et al. Survival after lumpectomy and mastectomy for early stage invasive breast cancer. *Cancer*, 2013;119:1402–1411.

59. Gottlieb S. Lumpectomy as good as mastectomy for tumors up to 5 cm across. *West J Med*. 2000;173(4):227-228.

60. Plesca M et al. Evolution of radical mastectomy for breast cancer. *J Med Life*. 2016;9(2):183–186.

61. The Complete Menopause Gallery, *Reader's Digest*. November 3, 2021. https://www.readersdigest.co.uk/health/wellbeing/the-complete-menopause-glossary

62. Chen Y et al. Midlife women's perceptions and attitudes about menopause. *Menopause*. 1998; 5(1): 28–34.

63. The North American Menopause Society. Menopause 101: A Primer for the Perimenopausal. https://www.menopause.org/for-women/menopauseflashes/meno-pause-symptoms-and-treatments/menopause-101-a-primer-for-the-perimenopausal. Accessed May 27, 2024.

64. Joffe H et al. Impact of estradiol variability and progesterone on mood in peri-menopausal women with depressive symptoms. *J Clin Endocrinol Metab*. 2020 Mar 1;105(3):e642–50. Accessed April 28, 2024.

65. Allen J et al. Needs assessment of menopause education in United States obstetrics and gynecology residency training programs. *Menopause*. 2023; 30(10): 1002–1005.

66. Monis C et al. Menstrual cycle proliferative and follicular phase. In: *StatPearls [Internet]*. Treasure Island (FL): StatPearls Publishing; 2024 Jan. Updated Sep 12, 2022. https://www.ncbi.nlm.nih.gov/books/NBK542229/. Accessed April 28, 2024.

67. Li D et al. The effect of menstrual cycle phases on approach-avoidance behaviors in women: evidence from conscious and unconscious processes. POctober 21, 2022. *Brain Sci*. 2022 Oct 21;12(10):1417. Accessed April 28, 2024.

68. Schleifenbaum L et al. Women feel more attractive before ovulation: evidence from a large-scale online diary study. September 1, 2021. *Evolutionary Human Sciences*. 2021;3:e47. Accessed April 28, 2024.

69. Nagy B et al. Key to life: physiological role and clinical implications of progesterone. October 13, 2021. *Int J Mol Sci*. 2021 Oct 13;22(20):11039. Accessed April 28, 2024.

70. Mitchell ES et al. Midlife women's attributions about perceived memory changes: observations from the Seattle midlife women's health study, *J Womens Health Gend Based Med,* 2001 10:4, 351–362.

71. Maki PM et al. Brain fog in menopause: a health-care professional's guide for decision-making and counseling on cognition. *Climacteric*. 2022; 25(6):5 70–578.

72. Keep P et al. The ageing woman. In: Lauritzen C., van Keep P.A., editors. *Ageing and Estrogens. Frontiers of Hormone Research,* Proceedings of the 1st International Workshop on Estrogen Therapy, Geneva, Switzerland, 1972. Volume 2. S. Karger; Basel, Switzerland: 1973. pp. 160–173.

73. Kopera H. The dawn of hormone replacement therapy. *Maturitas.* 1991 Sep; (3):187–188.

74. Michaleas S et al. Joseph Lister (1827–1912): A pioneer of antiseptic surgery. *Cureus.* December 21, 2022. 2022 Dec 21;14(12):e32777. Accessed April 28, 2024.

75. Vance D. Premarin: the intriguing history of a controversial drug. *Int J Pharm Compd.* 2007;1 1(4): 282–286.

76. Bell S. Sociological perspectives on the medicalization of menopause. *Annals of the New York Academy of Sciences,* 1990; 592(1): 173–178.

77. Smith D et al. Association of exogenous estrogen and endometrial carcinoma. *New England Journal of Medicine,* 1975; 293(23): 1164–1167.

78. Grady D et al. . Heart and Estrogen/progestin Replacement Study (HERS): design, methods, and baseline characteristics. *Control Clin Trials.* 1998;19(4):314–35.

79. North American Menopause Society. NAMS Position Statement Menopause: The 2022 Hormone Therapy Position Statement of the North American Menopause Society. Menopause. 2022;29(7):767–749.

80. Stuenkel C et al. Treatment of symptoms of the menopause: an endocrine society clinical practice guideline. *J Clin Endocrinol Metab.* 2015;100(11):3975–4011.

81. U.S. Food and Drug Administration. FDA Approves Novel Drug to Treat Moderate to Severe Hot Flashes Caused by Menopause. May 12, 2023. https://www .fda.gov/news-events/press-announcements/fda-approves-novel-drug-treat-moder-ate-severe-hot-flashes-caused-menopause#:~:text=Veozah percent20is percent20not percent20a percent20hormone,the percent20same percent20time percent20each percent20day.

82. National Institutes of Health. Black Cohosh. Updated June 3, 2020. https://ods .od.nih.gov/factsheets/BlackCohosh-HealthProfessional/. Accessed May 27, 2024.

83. Bedell S et al. The pros and cons of plant estrogens for menopause. *J Steroid Biochem Mol Biol.* 2014;139: 225–236.

84. Newson L et al. The dangers of compounded bioidentical hormone replacement therapy. *Br J Gen Pract.* 2019; 69(688): 540–541.

85. Yong E et al. Menopausal osteoporosis: screening, prevention and treatment. *Singapore Med J.* 2021; 62(4): 159–166.

86. Naumova I, Castelo-Branco C. Current treatment options for postmenopausal vaginal atrophy. *Int J Womens Health.* 2018; 10: 387–395.

87. McVicker L et al. Vaginal estrogen therapy use and survival in females with breast cancer. *JAMA Oncol.* 2024;10(1):103–108.

88. AARP. AARP Travel Research: Multi-Generational Travel. April 27, 2015. https://www.aarp.org/pri/topics/social-leisure/travel/aarp-travel-research-multi-gen-erational-travel.html.

89. Kumar A et al. Waiting for merlot: anticipatory consumption of experiential and material purchases. *Psychological Science* 25, no. 10 (October 2014): 1924–31.

90. Centers for Disease Control and Prevention. Emergency Department Visits. Reviewed April 15, 2024. https://www.cdc.gov/nchs/fastats/emergency-department .htm. Accessed May 27, 2024.

91. National Conference of State Legislatures. Map Monday: Rural Hospitals Closing Their Doors. Updated August 7, 2023. https://www.ncsl.org/resources/map -monday-rural-hospitals-closing-their-doors#:~:text=But percent20in percent20the percent20last percent2018,Center percent20for percent20Health percent20Services percent20Research. Accessed May 27, 2024.

92. Smalley C et al. The impact of hospital boarding on the emergency department waiting room. *J Am Coll Emerg Physicians Open.* 2020 May;1(5):1052–1059.

93. Resnick LA. Urgent Care: the evolution of a revolution. Published October 23, 2013. *Isr J Health Policy Res.* 2013 Oct 23;2(1):39. Accessed April 20, 2024.

94. Medline Plus. Recognizing Medical Emergencies, *MedlinePlus.* Reviewed January 2, 2023. https://medlineplus.gov/ency/article/001927.htm. Accessed May 27, 2024.

95. EMTALA and Prudent Layperson Standard FAQ, American College of Emergency Physicians. Updated May 2024. https://www.acep.org/administration /reimbursement/reimbursement-faqs/emtala-and-prudent-layperson-standard-faq. Accessed 27 May 2024.

96. Zupan Julie, Rabbi. What is the Jewish Expression to Refer to Someone Who Has Died? *Reform Judiasm,* https://reformjudaism.org/learning/answers-jewish -questions/what-jewish-expression-refer-someone-who-has-died. Accessed 27 May 2024.

CHAPTER 9

1. Nikolaeva E et al. The impact of daily affective touch on cortisol levels in institutionalized & fostered children. April 1, 2024, epub February 1, 2024. *Physiol Behav.* 2024 Apr 1;277:114479. doi: 10.1016/j.physbeh.2024.114479. PMID: 38309608. Accessed May 11, 2024.

2. Kertes D et al. Early deprivation and home basal cortisol levels: a study of internationally adopted children. *Dev Psychopathol.* 2008; 20(2): 473–491.

3. Wismer Fries A et al. Early experience in humans is associated with changes in neuropeptides critical for regulating social behavior. *Proc Natl Acad Sci* USA. 2005; 102(47): 17237–40.

4. Moore E et al. Early skin-to-skin contact for mothers and their healthy new-born infants. November 26, 2016. *Cochrane Database of Systematic Reviews*, 2016, Issue 11. Art. No.: CD003519. DOI: 10.1002/14651858.CD003519.pub4. Accessed May 11, 2024.

5. Widström A et al. Skin-to-skin contact the first hour after birth, underlying implications and clinical practice. *Acta Paediatr.* 2019; 108(7): 1192–1204.

6. Packheiser J et al. A systematic review and multivariate meta-analysis of the physical and mental health benefits of touch interventions. April 8, 2024. *Nat Hum Behav* (2024). https://doi.org/10.1038/s41562-024-01841-8. Accessed May 13, 2024.

7. Holt-Lunstad J et al. Social isolation and loneliness as medical issues. *N Engl J Med.* 2023; 388(3):1 93–195.

8. Pizzarro J. The efficacy of art and writing therapy: Increasing positive mental health outcomes and participant retention after exposure to a traumatic experience. *Art Therapy.* 2004; 21(1): 5–12.

9. Baikie K et al. Emotional and physical health benefits of expressive writing. *Adv in Psychiatr Treat.* 2005: 11(5): 338–346.

10. Koschwanez H et al. Expressive writing and wound healing in older adults: a randomized controlled trial. *Psychosom Med.* 2013; 75(6): 581–90.

11. Shimbo D. Translational research of the acute effects of negative emotions on vascular endothelial health: findings from a randomized controlled study, *JAHA,* 7 May 2024(13)9. https://www.ahajournals.org/doi/10.1161/JAHA.123.032698. Accessed June 7, 2024.

12. Kanaya Y et al. Anger is eliminated with the disposal of a paper written because of provocation. April 9, 2024. *Sci Rep* 14, 7490 (2024). https://doi.org/10 .1038/s41598-024-57916-z. Accessed May 13, 2024.

13. Welp L et al. Self-compassion, empathy and helping intentions. *J Posit Psychol.* 2014; 9(1): 54–65.

14. Craig G. What is EFT? Theory, science and uses. https://www.emofree.com/ eft-tutorial/tapping-basics/what-is-eft.html. Accessed June 7, 2024.

15. Longhurst J. Defining meridians: a modern basis of understanding. *JAMS.* 2010; 3(2): 67–74.

16. Ortner J. What is tapping? *The Tapping Solution.* https://www.thetappingsolu- tion.com/tapping-101/. Accessed June 7, 2024.

17. Dincer B et al. The effect of Emotional Freedom Techniques on nurses' stress, anxiety, and burnout levels during the COVID-19 pandemic: A randomized con- trolled trial. *Explore (NY).* 2021; 17(2): 109–114.

18. Patterson S. The effect of emotional freedom technique on stress and anxiety in nursing students: A pilot study. *Nurse Educ Today.* 2016; 40: 104–110.

19. Nelms J et al. A systematic review and meta-analysis of randomized and non- randomized trials of clinical Emotional Freedom Techniques (EFT) for the treatment of depression. *Explore (NY).* 2016; 12(6): 416–426.

20. Wati N et al. The effect of EFT (Emotional Freedom Technique) to the self- esteem among nurses. *Mal J Med Health Sci.* 1 2022; 8(SUPP2): 239–242.

21. Bach D et al. Clinical EFT (Emotional Freedom Techniques) improves mul- tiple physiological markers of health. February 19, 2019. *J Evid Based Integr Med.* 2019 Jan-Dec;24:2515690X18823691. doi: 10.1177/2515690X18823691. PMID: 30777453; PMCID: PMC6381429. Accessed May 13, 2024.

22. Zhuang Y et al. History of acupuncture research. *Int Rev Neurobiol.* 2013; 111: 1–23.

23. Cabyogly M et al. The mechanism of acupuncture. *Int J Neurosci.* 2005; 116(2): 115–125.

24. Hu B et al. The endocannabinoid system, a novel and key participant in acu- puncture's multiple beneficial effects. *Neurosci Biobehav Rev.* 2017; 77: 340–357.

25. Errington-Evans N. Acupuncture for anxiety. *CNS Neurosci Ther.* 2012; 18(4): 277–284.

26. Chae Y et al. Effect of acupuncture on anxiety-like behaviour during nicotine withdrawal and relevant mechanisms. *Neurosci Lett.* 2008; 430: 98–102.

27. Hollifield M et al. Acupuncture for posttraumatic stress disorder. *The J Nerv Ment Dis* 2007; 195: 504–513.

28. Wang S et al. Auricular acupuncture: a potential treatment for anxiety. *A & A.* 2001; 92(2): 548–553.

29. Amorim D et al. Acupuncture and electroacupuncture for anxiety disorders: A systematic review of the clinical research. *Complement Ther Clin Pract.* 2018; 31: 31–37.

30. Mills P et al. Beta-adrenergic receptor sensitivity in subjects practicing Transcendental Meditation. *J Psychosom Res.* 1990; 34: 29–33.

31. Ditto B et al. Short-term autonomic and cardiovascular effects of mindfulness body scan meditation, *Ann Behav Med.* 2006; 32(3): 227–234.

32. Brook R et al. Beyond medications and diet: Alternative approaches to lowering blood pressure: A scientific statement from the American Heart Association. *Hypertens.* 2013; 61:1360–83.

33. Jevning R et al. Adrenocortical activity during meditation. *Horm Behav.* 1978; 10(1): 54–60.

34. Hilton L et al. Mindfulness meditation for chronic pain: systematic Review and meta-analysis. *Ann Behav Med.* 2017; 51(2): 199–213.

35. Burns J et al. The effect of meditation on self -reported measures of stress, anxiety, depression and perfectionism in college population. *J Coll Stud Psych.* 2011; 25(2): 132–144.

36. Oman D et al. Meditation lowers stress and supports forgiveness among college students: a randomized controlled trial, *J Am Coll Health.* 2008; 58(5): 569–578.

37. Chen K et al. Meditative therapies for reducing anxiety: a systematic review and meta-analysis of randomized controlled trials. *Depress Anxiety.* 2012; 29(7): 545–562.

38. Orme-Johnson D et al. Effects of the transcendental meditation technique on trait anxiety: a meta-analysis of randomized controlled trials. *J Altern Complement Med.* 2014; 20(5): 330–341.

39. Rusch H et al. The effect of mindfulness meditation on sleep quality: a systematic review and meta-analysis of randomized controlled trials. *Ann N Y Acad Sci.* 2019; 1445(1): 5–16.

40. American Psychological Association. Stress in America: Paying with Our Health, American Psychological Association. February 4, 2015. https://www.apa.org /news/press/releases/stress/2014/stress-report.pdf. Accessed June 7 2024.

41. Kern M et al. Personality and pathway influence on health. *Soc Personal Psychol Compass.* 2011; 5(1): 76–87.

42. Steptoe A et al. Positive affect measured using ecological momentary assessment and survival in older men and women. *PNAS.* 2021; 108(45): 18244–18248.

43. Lozano M et al. Happiness and life expectancy by main occupational position among older workers: Who will live longer and happy? *SSM Popul Health.* 2021

Jan 14;13:100735. doi: 10.1016/j.ssmph.2021.100735. PMID: 33511266; PMCID: PMC7815996. Accessed June 1, 2024.

44. Konrath S et al. Motives for volunteering are associated with mortality risk in older adults. *Health Psychol.* 2012; 31(1): 87–96.

45. Mobbs D et al. The ecology of human fear: survival optimization and the nervous system. March 18, 2015. *Front Neurosci.* 2015 Mar 18;9:55. doi: 10.3389/fnins.2015.00055. PMID: 25852451; PMCID: PMC4364301. Accessed June 1, 2024.

46. Kendler K et al. Fears and phobias: reliability and heritability. *Psychol Med.* 1999; 29(3): 539–553.

47. Horikoshi K. The positive psychology of challenge: Towards interdisciplinary studies of activities and processes involving challenges. *Front Psychol.* 2023 Jan 13;13:1090069. doi: 10.3389/fpsyg.2022.1090069. PMID: 36743637; PMCID: PMC9891132. Accessed June 1, 2024.

48. Furmark T et al. Social phobia in the general population: prevalence and sociodemographic profile. *Soc Psychiatry Psychiatr Epidemiol.* 1999; 34(8): 416–24.

49. Henschke S. Why Are We Scared of Public Speaking? Psychology Today. November 2017. https://www.psychologytoday.com/us/blog/smashing-the-brain-blocks/201711/why-are-we-scared-of-public-speaking#:~:text=Fear percent20of percent20public percent20speaking percent20is percent20frequently percent20but percent20incorrectly percent20cited percent20as,of percent20people percent20report percent20experiencing percent20it.

50. Chandola T, Zhang N. Re-employment, job quality, health and allostatic load biomarkers: Prospective evidence from the UK Household Longitudinal Study. *Brain Behav Immun.* 2018;76:132–140. https://www.sciencedirect.com/science/article/abs/pii/S1472811719300497.

51. Toastmasters International, https://www.toastmasters.org. Accessed 7 June 2024.

52. Mindel N. King David. Chabad.org, https://www.chabad.org/library/article_cdo/aid/112317/jewish/King-David.htm#:~:text=Not percent20as percent20a percent20great percent20warrior,The percent20Sweetest percent20Poetry percent20of percent20Israel. Accessed 7 June 2024.

53. Andrade C et al. Prayer and healing: A medical and scientific perspective on randomized controlled trials. *Indian J Psychiatry.* 2009; 51(4): 247–253.

54. Romez C et al. Case report of gastroparesis healing: 16 years of a chronic syndrome resolved after proximal intercessory prayer. *Complement Ther Med.* 2019; 43: 289–294.

55. Leibovici L. Effects of remote, retroactive intercessory prayer on outcomes in patients with bloodstream infection: randomised controlled trial. *BMJ.* 2001; 323: 1450–1451.

56. cdc.gov. About Mental Health, U.S. Centers for Disease Control and Prevention. Last Reviewed 16 April 2024. https://www.cdc.gov/mentalhealth/learn/index.htm#:~:text=How percent20common percent20are percent20mental percent20illnesses,a percent20seriously percent20debilitating percent20mental percent20illness. Accessed 7 June 2024.

57. National Institute of Mental Health. Women and mental health, National Institute of Mental Health, https://www.nimh.nih.gov/health/topics/women-and-mental-health. Accessed 7 June 2024.

58. Nicks B et al. The impact of psychiatric patient boarding in emergency departments. July 12, 2012. *Emerg Med Int.* 2012;2012:360308. doi: 10.1155/2012/360308. Epub 2012 Jul 22. PMID: 22888437; PMCID: PMC3408670.

59. Chang B et al. The depressed patient and suicidal patient in the emergency department: evidence-based management and treatment strategies. *Emerg Med Pract.* 2011;13 (9): 1–23.

60. Beck A. Cognitive therapy: nature and relation to behavior therapy. *Behav. Ther.* 1970; 1(2): 184–200.

61. Beck JS et al. A brief history of Aaron T. Beck, MD, and cognitive behavior therapy. June 18 ,2021. *Clin Psychol Eur.* 2021 Jun 18;3(2):e6701. doi: 10.32872/cpe.6701. PMID: 36397957; PMCID: PMC9667129.. Accessed June 2 2024.

62. Hofmann S et al. The efficacy of cognitive behavioral therapy: a review of meta-analyses. *Cognit Ther Res.* 2012; 36(5): 427–440.

63. Hasler G. Pathophysiology of depression: do we have any solid evidence of interest to clinicians? *World Psychiatry.* 2010; 9(3): 155–161.

64. Hofmann S et al. Is it beneficial to add pharmacotherapy to cognitive behavioral therapy when treating anxiety disorders? A meta-analytic review. *Int J Cogn Ther.* 2009; 2(2):160–175.

65. Scherma M et al. Brain activity of anandamide: a rewarding bliss? *Acta Pharmacol Sin.* 2019; 40(3): 309–323.

66. Baggalar M. 2-Arachidonoylglycerol: A signaling lipid with manifold actions in the brain. *Prog. Lipid Res.*2018; 71: 1–17.

67. Kibret B et al. Crosstalk between the endocannabinoid and mid-brain dopaminergic systems: Implication in dopamine dysregulation. *Front Behav Neurosci.* 2023 Mar 16;17:1137957. doi: 10.3389/fnbeh.2023.1137957. PMID: 37009000; PMCID: PMC10061032.

68. Lichenstein S. THC, CBD, and Anxiety: A review of recent findings on the anxiolytic and anxiogenic effects of cannabis' primary cannabinoids. *Curr Addict Rep.* 2022; 9(4): 473–485.

69. Zuardi AW et al. Action of cannabidiol on the anxiety and other effects produced by delta 9-THC in normal subjects. *Psychopharmacol (Berl).* 1982;76(3):245–50.

70. The Food and Drug Administration. FDA warns patients and health care providers about potential risks associated with compounded ketamine products, including oral formulations, for the treatment of psychiatric disorders. October 10, 2023. https://www.fda.gov/drugs/human-drug-compounding/fda-warns-patients-and-health-care-providers-about-potential-risks-associated-compounded-ketamine. Accessed 7 June 2024.

71. The Food and Drug Administration. FDA approves new nasal spray medication for treatment-resistant depression; available only at certified doctor's office or clinic. March 5, 2019. https://www.fda.gov/news-events/press-announcements/fda-approves-new-nasal-spray-medication-treatment-resistant-depression-available-only-certified. Accessed 7 June 2024.

72. Zanos P et al. Mechanisms of ketamine action as an antidepressant. *Mol Psychiatry.* 2018; 23(4): 801–811.

73. Matveychuk D et al. Ketamine as an antidepressant: overview of its mechanisms of action and potential predictive biomarkers. May 11, 2020. *Ther Adv Psychopharmacol.* 2020 May 11;10:2045125320916657. doi: 10.1177/2045125320916657. PMID: 32440333; PMCID: PMC7225830. Accessed June 2, 2024.

74. Henderson T. Practical application of the neuroregenerative properties of ketamine: real world treatment experience. *Neural Regen Res* 2016; 11: 195–200.

75. Mandal S et al. Efficacy of ketamine therapy in the treatment of depression. *Indian J Psychiatry.* 2019; 61(5): 480–485.

76. Rizvi S et al. Use of transcranial magnetic stimulation for depression. May 23, 2019. *Cureus.* 2019 May 23;11(5):e4736. doi: 10.7759/cureus.4736. PMID: 31355095; PMCID: PMC6649915. Accessed June 2, 2024.

77. Carmi L et al. Efficacy and safety of deep transcranial magnetic stimulation for obsessive-compulsive disorder: A prospective multicenter randomized double-blind placebo-controlled trial. *Am J Psychiatry.* 2019;1 76(11): 931–938.

78. Roth Y et al. Real-world efficacy of deep TMS for obsessive-compulsive disorder: post-marketing data collected from twenty-two clinical sites. *J of Psych Res.* 2020; 137: 667–672.

79. Gunther M et al. Cranial electrotherapy stimulation for the treatment of depression. *J. Psychosoc. Nurs. Ment. Health Serv.* 2010; 48: 37–42.

80. Bracciano A et al. Cranial electrotherapy stimulation in the treatment of posttraumatic stress disorder: a pilot study of two military veterans. *J. Neurother.* 2012; 16: 60–69.

81. Morriss R et al. Differential effects of cranial electrotherapy stimulation on changes in anxiety and depression symptoms over time in patients with generalized anxiety disorder. *J. Affect. Disord.* 2020; 277:785–788.

82. Karlović D et al. Eighty years of ECT in Croatia and in Sestre Milosrdnice University Hospital Center. *Acta Clin Croat.* 2020; 59(3): 489–495.

83. Singh A et al. How electroconvulsive therapy works? Understanding the neurobiological mechanisms. *Clin Psychopharmacol Neurosci.* 2017; 15(3):2 10–221.

84. Baghai TC et al. Electroconvulsive therapy and its different indications. *Dialogues Clin Neurosci.* 2008; 10(1): 105–117.

CHAPTER 10

1. Mohr T. Why women don't apply for jobs unless 100 percent qualified. HBR. August 25, 2014. https://hbr.org/2014/08/why-women-dont-apply-for-jobs-unless -theyre-100-qualified . Accessed June 12, 2024.

Index

AARP, 110
abdominal fat, 41, 73
active lifestyle, 72. *See also* exercise
acupuncture, 121–123
addiction. *See* substance use and abuse
ADHD (attention deficit hyperactivity disorder), 76
adrenaline and adrenal glands, xviii, 4, 5, 63, 74. *See also* fight-or-flight response
Affordable Care Act (2010), 111
aging: acceptance and, 14, 49–50; attitude and mental health, 14; exercise and, 54, 73; facial appearance and, 61, 91–92; physical appearance as indicator of health, 50–51, 109 ; premature, 54, 94; preparing for, 91–95; sex and, 74; telomere length and, 33; yo-yo dieting and, 90
alcohol. *See* substance use and abuse
American Cancer Society, 97
American College of Emergency Physicians, 7, 112
American Heart Association (AHA), 77, 96, 97, 98
American Medical Association (AMA), 43

American Psychological Association, 82, 124
American Public Health Association, 81–82
amygdala, 4–5, 80, 123
anandamide, 8, 9, 66, 73, 131
anger and hostility, 5, 14, 46, 63, 120
anorexia nervosa, 53
ANS (autonomic nervous system), 4–5, 93, 123
antidepressants, 9, 16, 45, 94, 130
anxiety: acupuncture for, 122–123; baths for, 70; cancer and, 14; career and, 21–22, 45; chronic stress and, 5; COVID-19 pandemic and, 17–18; debt and, 81–82; endocannabinoid system and, 131; exercise for, 71, 92; heart attacks and, 99; hoarding and, 67; journaling for, 120; laughter for, 66; loneliness and, 71; medications and treatments for, 9, 14, 16, 121–123, 128–130, 131–133; meditation for, 123; memory and, 107; nature and, 69; pet ownership for, 77; self-esteem and, 61, ; social media use and, 17; substance use and abuse, 83
2-Arachidonoylglycerol (2AG), 8, 73, 131
Archives of Internal Medicine, 63

About the Author

Dr. Leigh Vinocur, television's beloved medical analyst, is a board-certified emergency physician, prominent medical advisor in the corporate and industry healthcare sectors, and national spokesperson for the American College of Emergency Physicians. Dr. Leigh began her medical career as a pioneering woman in urology as the first women ever accepted to her residency program, prior to her emergency medicine residency. She also got one of the first master's degrees in the country in medical cannabis science and therapeutics. She was recently appointed by Governor Wes Moore of Maryland and serves on the state's Cannabis Public Health Advisory Council. As a medical physician executive, she has served as chief medical director running the 15 urgent care clinics, overseeing 150 clinicians serving over 150,000 patients per year. She has served as a chief medical officer in the biotech and nutraceutical industries. With more than 30 years of experience as an emergency physician, she has become a fascinating, humorous medical expert on a variety of health and medical subjects.

A prominent member of the Dr. Oz Show's inaugural Medical Advisory Board, Dr. Leigh has been asked for medical advice by virtually every national television network and cable news outlet. She started as a consultant and medical reporter for Baltimore's NBC affiliate, WBAL-TV, and the *NBC News Channel*. She became a familiar voice on WBAL radio Monday mornings with Dave Durian. From there, Dr. Leigh has become one of the go-to medical analysts including regular appearances on the popular syndicated *NewsNation Now, The Today Show,* the Fox News Channel, CNN's *House Calls* and the *Nancy Grace Show, HLN Prime News, The Dr. Oz Show, Inside Edition*, as well as *ABC News* and the *CBS Early Show*. She co-hosted a miniseries on alternative medicine with Dr. Kevin Soden on Comcast's Retirement Living Network. She has contributed health columns for the *Huffington*

Post, *Examiner* newspaper chain, Savvy Auntie, and the Dr. Oz website as one of their medical experts. She writes a column for the Hearst publication, GreenState.com called "Ask Dr. Leigh," where she answers readers' questions on medical cannabis. Additionally, she has been profiled in feature article in the magazine *More* called, "This Is What 50 Looks Like."

www.ingramcontent.com/pod-product-compliance
Lightning Source LLC
LaVergne TN
LVHW021200160725
816212LV00002BA/192